Case
Studies in
Emergency
Medicine

Case Studies in Emergency Medicine

Frederic W. Platt, M.D., F.A.C.P.
Clinical Assistant Professor of Medicine,
University of Colorado School of Medicine;
Director of Medicine, Presbyterian Medical Center;
Attending Physician, Emergency Department,
Denver General Hospital, Denver

Little, Brown and Company, Boston

93301

To the many patients
who trust us
when they are so much
in need of help

Preface

THE CASES IN THIS COLLECTION exemplify some of the more common problems seen in the emergency room of a busy city hospital. Some are of a serious nature, while others are seemingly trivial. Some demonstrate good medical care, but many were selected because they show errors of diagnosis or management. The discussions are intended for the student, physician, nurse, or paramedic working in the emergency room. All cases are real and unaltered.

The cases are randomly arranged, just as patients arrive at the emergency room without grouping by disease or by physician's specialty. The selection features the acutely ill patient rather than the trauma patient, reflecting our emergency room patient load (70% nontrauma). Many surgical textbooks cover the management of the trauma patient well, and the therapeutic approach to trauma is relatively well worked out. The approach to many medical emergencies and urgencies has not been clearly formulated.

The cases were chosen from among those seen at Denver General Hospital and the management discussions represent approaches we presently use. In many situations, the correct management is not really known, and the course suggested in this book can be viewed only as our present choice in a nebulous area. The cases we see are heavily weighted by several factors that do not apply in all emergency rooms. Over 50% of our patients have alcohol as one of the causes of their visits to the emergency room (intoxicated, withdrawing, in auto accident hit by a drunk driver, etc.). Most emergency patients using city ambulances are brought to our hospital. This gives us a high fraction of true emergencies and a high fraction of destitute, homeless, and familyless patients.

Denver General Hospital has a small number of inpatient beds for a city of its size, so we are obliged to refuse admission to many patients who would be best dealt with by a 24- to 48-hour inpatient stay, thus tending to prolong their stay in the emergency room proper. We have no holding ward for observation cases, brief stay cases, or "precoronary care" cases. This, too, tends to increase the length of time patients spend in the emergency room. In a hospital with a large observation unit or more inpatient beds for a comparable population, more patients could quickly leave the emergency room, and much of the management described in this text could take place elsewhere in the hospital.

Many of the cases described will seem unfinished. The reader will probably wonder what happened to the patient after he left the emergency room. Unfortunately, this sense of unfinished business is frequently found in emergency-room work. The physician often loses contact with the patient and is left wondering just what became of him. While this is not optimal, it is common and is demonstrated in some of these cases.

Since the cases in this book are arranged randomly, a reader who wishes to read cases relating to a specific problem must make use of the index.

Case Studies in Emergency Medicine is intended not to replace but to supplement standard textbooks on emergency medicine and surgery. Any emergency room should have on hand at least a minimal collection of reference books. Some that we have found useful are:

Wintrobe, M. W., et al. (Eds.). *Harrison's Principles of Internal Medicine,* 6th ed. New York: McGraw-Hill, 1970.

Gleason, M. N., et al. *Clinical Toxicology of Commercial Products.* Baltimore: Williams & Wilkins, 1969.

Goodman, L. S., and Gilman, A. (Eds.). *The Pharmacological Basis of Therapeutics,* 4th ed. New York: Macmillan, 1970.

Plum, F., and Posner, J. B. *The Diagnosis of Stupor and Coma,* 2nd ed. Philadelphia: Davis, 1972.

Lockhart, R. D., Hamilton, G. F., and Fyfe, F. W. *Anatomy of the Human Body.* Philadelphia: Lippincott, 1969.

Williamson, P. *Office Procedures,* 2nd ed. Philadelphia: Saunders, 196

American Hospital Formulary Service. *Hospital Formulary.* Washington, D.C.: American Society of Hospital Pharmacists, 1971.

Physicians' Desk Reference, 27th ed. Oradell, N.J.: Medical Economics Co., 1973.

Bailey, H. *Demonstrations of Physical Signs in Clinical Surgery,* 13th ed. Baltimore: Williams & Wilkins, 1960.

Merritt, H. *A Textbook of Neurology,* 5th ed. Philadelphia: Lea & Febiger, 1970.

American College of Surgeons, Committee on Trauma. *Early Care of the Injured Patient.* Philadelphia: Saunders, 1972.

Shires, G. T. (Ed.). *Care of the Trauma Patient.* New York: McGraw-Hill, 1966.

Ballinger, W. F., Rutherford, R. B., and Zuidema, G. D. *The Management of Trauma.* Philadelphia: Saunders, 1968.

Schneewind, J. H. (Ed.). *Medical and Surgical Emergencies.* Chicago: Year Book, 1968.

Eckert, C. (Ed.). *Emergency-Room Care,* 2d ed. Boston: Little, Brown, 1971.

Moore, M. E. (Ed.). *Medical Emergency Manual.* Baltimore: Williams & Wilkins, 1972.

Murphy, F. D. *Medical Emergencies: Diagnosis and Treatment.* Philadelphia: Davis, 1958.

Ellis, M. *The Casualty Officer's Handbook,* 3d ed. London: Butterworth, 1970.

Washington University Department of Medicine. *Manual of Medical Therapeutics,* 20th ed. Edited by M. G. Rosenfeld. Boston: Little, Brown, 1971.

Driesbach, R. H. *Handbook of Poisoning: Diagnosis and Treatment.* Los Altos, Calif.: Lange, 1971.

Kaye, S. *Handbook of Emergency Toxicology,* 3d ed. Springfield, Ill.: Thomas, 1970.

Thienes, C. H., and Haley, T. J. *Clinical Toxicology,* 5th ed. Philadelphia: Lea & Febiger, 1972.

Tynes, J. H., and Sutherland, J. M. *Exercises in Neurological Diagnosis.* London: Livingstone, 1967.

Numerous journals contain articles pertinent to emergency work. Several frequently include useful studies. It would be reasonable for a well-equipped emergency room to carry recent issues of the following:

The Journal of Trauma
The Journal of the American Medical Association
The Annals of Internal Medicine
Emergency Medicine
Journal of the American College of Emergency Physicians
Clinical Toxicology
The Medical Letter
Clinical Pharmacology and Therapeutics

Acknowledgments

THIS BOOK would not have been written without a great deal of help from friends and associates. Many of the physicians at Denver General Hospital contributed their thoughts and moral support. Especially helpful were Drs. Peter Bryson, Robert Elliott, Gerald Gordon, Warren Hern, Roger Johnson, Paul Lessig, Avrum Organick, J. C. Owens, Cleve Trimble, William Turner, and Philip Yarnell. Ms. Marilynn Webb and Ms. Consuela Quintana were indefatigable in their secretarial assistance. The initial and final versions were edited by my wife Constance. Ms. Phyllis H. Ehrlich of Little, Brown and Company supervised the editorial production of the book.

Contents

Case
Studies in
Emergency
Medicine

A 40-YEAR-OLD MAN was brought to the emergency room by
ambulance. He claimed to have been assaulted by several men and
beaten about the chest and abdomen. On arrival he complained of
severe abdominal pain.

On examination, his supine pulse and blood pressure were 90
and 140/80, respectively. Sitting and then standing briefly led
to a pulse and blood pressure of 100 and 120/80. His chest was
clear to auscultation, but bilateral lower chest tenderness was
noted. There was no evidence of head trauma, his fundi showed
no hemorrhages, and his tympanic membranes were normal. His
abdomen was diffusely tender and showed rigid guarding throughout. When his attention was distracted, his abdomen could be
palpated fairly deeply without causing noticeable pain. Bowel
sounds were infrequent but present. Rectal examination was unremarkable, although the patient claimed not to enjoy the procedure.

What is the likelihood that this patient has a serious intra-
abdominal injury: perforation of bowel, tear of viscera, or other
problem requiring laparotomy?

What further studies should be done?

Can we send the patient home?

1 DISCUSSION

This patient seems to have no serious damage. The seriousness of blunt abdominal or chest trauma is, however, easy to underestimate. All such patients should be approached as potential fatalities. The major problem is occult intra-abdominal bleeding.

If the emergency declares itself by a low blood pressure, and if ventilation and oxygenation are adequate, then vigorous intravenous fluid therapy is needed. If the blood pressure responds to fluids (saline solution, lactated Ringer's solution, blood, etc.) then one may occasionally temporize, but in general, surgery is appropriate. One should operate freely, since the degree of intra-abdominal visceral damage often far exceeds what is initially apparent in blunt trauma.

If the blood pressure and pulse are not worrisome, then a tilt test (sitting, then standing the patient) should be done. As a simple rule of thumb, a pulse rise of at least 30 beats per minute or a mean blood pressure drop of at least 15 mm Hg suggests hypovolemia. (Of course, other processes involving drugs, sepsis, or hypoxia can also lead to such signs.)

The patient who has no signs of hypovolemia but who has significant blunt trauma (a human fist blow can result in a torn spleen or liver) should be observed in the hospital at least overnight. We usually use an abdominal tap as well. Our procedure is to insert a large (14-gauge) intracatheter through the midline — linea alba — about 1 to 2 cm below the umbilicus. Normal saline solution, 1000 ml, is then run in rapidly, and the bottle is disconnected from the intracatheter, which, still inserted, is allowed to drain freely onto a clean 4 X 4 gauze pad. Most observers can detect a pink color to the returning fluid when blood is present in a concentration of less than 0.1 ml blood per liter of returning fluid. The bladder should be decompressed with a Foley catheter prior to the abdominal tap. A midline scar from prior surgery may interfere with this diagnostic procedure. A woman usually accumulates free blood low in the pelvis, so a simple needling of the posterior vaginal cul-de-sac will work as well as an abdominal tap in finding free blood. In general, if the tap shows free blood, the patient should be explored. There is a small incidence of false positive and false negative taps.

This patient had an abdominal tap (it proved negative) and lavage, and spent an uneventful twenty-four hours in the hospital before being discharged.

2

A 19-YEAR-OLD WOMAN came to the emergency room complaining of having been fatigued for several weeks. She denied fever, pains, shortness of breath, cough, and bleeding. She felt she was operating at about 50% of her usual energy.

She had one child, a 6-month-old boy, and was working part-time as a file clerk. She described her relationship with her husband as being "good and bad" but denied being depressed. She denied using drugs of any sort.

On physical examination, she had a temperature of 37.4°C (99.2°F) and shotty cervical lymph adenopathy. She had a palpable spleen tip, according to one of two examiners. The rest of the findings were thought to be within normal limits.

What are the most common causes of fatigue in a young adult?

Do any of these represent true medical emergencies?

Can you prescribe a tonic for her?

Fatigue is one of the least directive symptoms — that is, it leads least well to any precise diagnosis. In a young person, the first causes of fatigue to consider are boredom, depression, true physical overwork, or a combination of these. After these, one must consider infections, for acute illnesses such as mononucleosis and hepatitis often present with pronounced fatigue as an outstanding symptom. Finally, tumor disease or failure of any major organ system can produce fatigue. Heart failure, respiratory insufficiency, renal failure, or anemia should be considered. Such a major system failure is an uncommon cause of fatigue in youth but is much more common in older adults. True medical emergencies may occur in organ system failure, but a more common emergency is the depressed and suicidal patient who presents with organic symptoms and may at first deny psychopathology.

Drug abuse, common among young adults, may cause fatigue, or associated illnesses such as hepatitis may do so. The examiner must use the correct contemporary terminology in questioning such patients, for a patient who denies drug use may admit to use of analgesics, sedatives, tranquilizers, birth control pills, and laxatives. A patient who denies "taking medicines" may admit to "popping" or "shooting up." One should be alert to the housewife syndrome of "alternating uppers and downers."

The patient described has some features suggestive of a viral illness such as mononucleosis. There is no apparent urgency to her problem. Fatigue in a young person is seldom an emergency except as a sign of suicidal depression.

It would be appropriate to obtain certain laboratory studies, such as a chest x-ray, urinalysis, biochemical survey (for hepatic enzymes, bilirubin, BUN, etc.), complete blood count, and mononucleosis spot test. She could be told to return for reevaluation in two to three days, at which time the laboratory results should be available. No therapy need be initiated. It should be clearly explained to the patient that correct therapy must await correct diagnosis. Too often patients are sent home without therapy, and they fail to understand that the doctor must know what he is treating before he prescribes treatment for it. This principle should be explained to the patient.

There is no broad-spectrum tonic available, despite popular belief to the contrary. This point also may need to be discussed with a patient who expects vitamins or some other "energy tonic."

3

AN 18-YEAR-OLD MAN came to the emergency room following an auto accident. His car had hit a tree, and his forehead hit the windshield, lacerating his right brow. Because of crowded conditions in the emergency room, he was seen only briefly by a nurse and then obliged to wait almost two hours before a physician could suture his wound. At the time of treatment, he claimed he felt fine, although he had been rather tired while waiting and appreciated the chance to rest. A cursory neurologic examination revealed no abnormalities. His laceration was debrided, cleaned, and sutured with 5-0 nylon. His eyebrow was not shaved. Because his last tetanus toxoid had been at age 8, he was given 0.5 ml of tetanus toxoid. The sutures were removed four days later, and his wound had healed well.

Four months later the man returned to the emergency room in the company of his mother. She claimed that he had been passing out since his injury. He had had about six episodes during which he stopped all activity, stared at the floor for several minutes, and once or twice fell to the floor. There were no associated involuntary movements and no incontinence. On close questioning, the patient recalled having a few spells during the year preceding his auto accident. He could not recall the exact events of his accident and never had been aware of striking the tree. After a faint, he usually would be a bit fatigued and sometimes momentarily confused. He denied dizziness, headache, or other symptoms. A thorough neurologic examination showed nothing abnormal, and there was no change of pulse or blood pressure when he changed from recumbent to standing position.

What is the matter with this young man?

Was his initial therapy correct?

What studies should be done?

The situation surrounding an accident may be of more importance than the event itself. It is possible that a more prompt physician evaluation of the young man described here might have revealed significant confusion and lethargy, pointing to preexisting neurologic disease or concussion. The past history regarding lapses of consciousness is pertinent.

In any case, the subsequent emergency-room visit suggests that the patient is having recurrent losses of consciousness and that a seizure disorder may be present. An EEG and skull films would be appropriate, and he deserves a followup evaluation by a neurologist. Following severe head trauma, the patient frequently complains of dull headaches, light-headedness, malaise, and depression, especially if he lost consciousness (had a concussion). He usually does not lose consciousness but often feels faint on rising rapidly. He may have retrograde amnesia for the accident itself, so this patient's failure to recall the accident precisely need not imply a seizure prior to the crash. Fainting spells or simple vasovagal syncope are common in otherwise well young men or women, but on awakening the patient is usually alert and not confused. Syncope seldom occurs when a patient is seated unless it is caused by an arrhythmia.

The initial treatment of this patient's laceration was correct. Some authorities believe that eyebrows may be shaved with impunity, but we usually do not do so. If shaved, the eyebrow may not grow back normally. If no tetanus toxoid had ever been given to the patient, he would have been given 250 units of human tetanus immune globulin followed by a tetanus toxoid immunization program. When a patient has received tetanus immunization within the last ten years, a booster dose of toxoid will call forth an adequate amnestic response.

4

AN 18-YEAR-OLD WOMAN was brought into the emergency room in a wheelchair. She had been assisted from a car and into the chair, but by the end of her 100-foot ride into the emergency room, she had stopped breathing and her color was blue-gray. A pulse was present, although thready, and her pulse rate was about 80. She was lifted onto a bed and began to vomit thin, green liquid. Her head was turned to the side and her pharynx suctioned with a tonsil-sucker. An oral airway was placed, and her lungs were ventilated with a self-inflating bag for about a minute while one of the doctors readied an endotracheal tube and a laryngoscope. When he was ready, the bag was removed and he succeeded in placing an oral tube in her trachea within one minute. If it had taken over one minute, the resuscitation chief would have terminated the attempt and returned to the Ambu bag.

A nurse spoke with the patient's friend who had brought her to the emergency department, and obtained information that the patient might have taken an overdose of propoxyphene (Darvon). A 5-mg dose of nalorphine was given intravenously. The patient had a minor motor seizure involving face and arms lasting one to two minutes. An intravenous infusion of 5% dextrose in water was started. Four more brief seizures followed. Ventilation continued with a self-inflating bag attached to the endotracheal tube, and another 5-mg dose of nalorphine was given intravenously ten minutes after the first dose. The patient's breathing returned, and her color improved. A Foley catheter was placed in her bladder, and 300 ml of urine was sent to the lab for toxicology study. A blood sample was drawn (with H_2O_2, rather than isopropyl alcohol, used to scrub the skin) and sent to the laboratory for alcohol, barbiturate, glucose, BUN, and electrolyte analyses and for CBC. A portable chest film was obtained, and a brief examination was made for neurologic and other major abnormalities. An esophageal tube (large-bore, Ewald-type) was placed in the stomach, and the patient was lavaged with 2000 ml of tap water in 400-ml amounts. The endotracheal tube cuff was inflated during all these events.

The patient was transferred to the medical intensive care unit within one hour of her arrival at the emergency room. While she was being transferred to a cart for the trip to the intensive care unit, a marijuana cigarette fell out of the pocket of her jacket. She awoke 6 hours later and admitted to taking about 60 Darvon capsules, 65 mg each.

Her emergency-room visit required the attention of three physicians and two nurses.

What are the most urgent activities in an overdose case such as this?

What do the seizures suggest?

Was the nalorphine the only therapeutic maneuver responsible for her improvement?

4 DISCUSSION

Amazingly, a fair number of patients seem to make it to the door of the emergency room and expire there. This patient was clearly dying on arrival. Only rapid, vigorous, knowledgeable, and well-coordinated care could help her. A ten-minute delay for a few small errors would have been fatal.

This patient arrived in acute brain and respiratory failure. The only appropriate therapy was to secure control of her airway and ventilate her. The airway is best controlled via an endotracheal tube, and a self-inflating bag is best for ventilation.

Emesis with aspiration is an ever-present danger during resuscitation and can be adequately guarded against only by obstructing the trachea with a cuffed tube. However, intubation will take seconds to minutes, and ventilation usually should be obtained first with a face mask. The physician intubator must ready all his equipment: laryngoscope, endotracheal tube and stylet and lubricant, syringe and clamp to inflate the cuff, and connectors for attachment of the tube to his source of ventilation, such as a self-inflating bag. Once he is ready, his operation must be timed by the resuscitation director, for the intubator will never be able to pay adequate attention to the amount of time he is taking during which the patient is not being ventilated. An independent physician must be willing to halt the intubation attempt and return to the mask after one minute and then reattempt intubation following several more minutes of ventilation. Of course, if adequate ventilation cannot be achieved with an Ambu bag and face mask, intubation must proceed and cannot be put off even these few minutes.

Seizures in an overdose patient are often the result of hypoxia. Certain drugs are notorious for causing seizures, even in the absence of hypoxia. These include Darvon, meperidine, antidepressants, anticholinergics, and antihistamines. Hypoglycemia should also be considered. A bolus of 50% glucose solution (50 ml) given intravenously is almost entirely safe in any comatose patient. Persistent seizures can be treated with anticonvulsants, but one should be hesitant to add further CNS sedatives to a comatose patient.

Nalorphine (Nalline) or naloxone (Narcan) is very effective in reversing narcotics overdose effects. They are less effective against Darvon than against heroin but still often are helpful. When treating patients with narcotics overdoses, one must be aware that the duration of action of heroin or other narcotics is far greater than the duration of action of any available narcotic antagonist. A patient may wake up, pull out his endotracheal tube, talk to his attendant, and then return to coma and hypoventilation as the antagonist wears off.

Any patient who has become hypoxic will be more obtunded than warranted by just the CNS depressive effect of the overdose drug. We have found that such patients respond well to ventilation for five to ten minutes. Thus, ventilation alone may return the patient to a state where he can adequately carry on ventilation thereafter. This makes the effect of the narcotic antagonist harder to evaluate. Naloxone (Narcan) is now available and being used in 0.4-mg doses that are repeatable every five to ten minutes. Naloxone has the benefit of *not* producing respiratory depression by itself, if indeed the case is not one of narcotics overdose.

Darvon, like heroin, may produce acute pulmonary edema. This condition may not be associated with a rising central venous pressure and may not respond to naloxone or nalorphine. One must listen to the patient's chest during ventilation and use x-ray technique to watch for this complication.

This patient might well have aspirated vomitus early in the resuscitation. Treatment should have included a large bolus of steroids (e.g., 1.0 gm of hydrocortisone) given intravenously.

5

TWELVE MEN from a fire department company were brought into the emergency room at 7 A.M. complaining of shortness of breath and coughing. They had responded to a call of chlorine gas escaping from a refrigeration and ice factory. The fire engine drove into the chlorine cloud, and before the crewmen could put on gas masks, they were all coughing and gasping.

The following describes events for a representative patient on arrival at the emergency room. The patient was a 35-year-old man who smoked two packs of cigarettes a day and had a mild persistent "cigarette cough." On this day he had had about five minutes of exposure to a thin chlorine cloud. On arrival, he was coughing and felt that he could not take a deep breath without triggering a paroxysm of coughing. A physical exam showed he was afebrile; pulse 100, respiratory rate 20, blood pressure 140/84. He was not cyanotic and appeared in little distress except that a deep breath brought on about twenty seconds of coughing. His chest revealed diffuse coarse wheezes with no rales. The cardiovascular examination was normal, and he had a normal pulmonic second sound. His initial therapy consisted of 1 gm of hydrocortisone intravenously, oxygen administered nasally, and 500 mg of aminophylline by rectal suppository. X-rays indicated a normal chest. After four hours in the emergency room, the patient felt a bit better and was sent home with instructions to return if he felt worse.

What are the dangers of toxic gas exposure?

What other tests might help decide the disposition of this case?

How is smoke inhalation related to this case?

The major problem in dealing with toxic gas exposure is that a sizable fraction of exposed cases may have only a mild bronchitis early but will later develop pulmonary edema. Usually this will occur within twenty-four hours of exposure if it is going to happen at all. Optimal management of this patient would include observation overnight, but if a place and persons are available outside to observe the patient, he may be sent out after four to eight hours with instructions to return if his breathing or coughing seems to be getting worse. An arterial blood gas analysis may help in making the decision.

Exposure to a chlorine cloud for five minutes is fatal to about one in a thousand victims, and the fatality rate is proportionately higher with longer exposures. The patient suffers bronchial spasm and cough. Later, alveolar changes and pulmonary capillary dilatation lead to chemical pulmonary edema, which can be treated with O_2, intermittent positive pressure breathing treatments, diuretics, aminophylline, steroids, or morphine, but not digitalis.

Chlorine gas and smoke are the two most common noxious inhalants that bring patients to the emergency room. The dose of noxious gas received should be estimated from the patient history. Smoke exposure may also be estimated by determining the venous blood carboxyhemoglobin level. If carbon monoxide binds less than 10% of the patient's hemoglobin and the patient is less than an hour from the time of exposure, one can usually assume that he received a fairly small dose and probably will not suffer severe delayed pulmonary effects. Chlorine does not leave such a measurable marker. In any case, an arterial blood-gas analysis will be helpful in evaluating oxygenation by the lungs. The arterial oxygen saturation is measured by a colorimetric technique and will read falsely high in a patient with smoke inhalation and carboxyhemoglobin. The pO_2 will, however, be accurate. Be sure the lab is measuring both pO_2 and oxygen saturation, and not just calculating one from the other.

6

A 30-YEAR-OLD MAN came to the emergency room at 2 A.M. complaining of pain and swelling in his left knee for several hours. He had previously been well, although on careful questioning he admitted to having had some burning on urination for a few days about two weeks earlier. He recalled no trauma to the knee and was on no medications.

Physical examination revealed that the patient had a warm, slightly erythematous, swollen left knee. The knee was tender, and attempts at flexion led to severe pain. All his other joints seemed normal. His conjunctiva were normal, and he had no urethral discharge. He had no heart murmur, no skin rash, no adenopathy, and no hepatosplenomegaly. He had no nodules, tophi, or other lumps, and was afebrile.

He was given codeine for his pain and referred to the arthritis clinic in two days.

Is acute monarticular arthritis ever an emergency?

Would you advise any laboratory studies?

Is there any danger in handling this case in this fashion?

There are few true rheumatologic emergencies. An acute non-traumatic monarticular arthritis is one of these. If the patient has not traumatized the joint by twisting, falling, or hitting it, and if he is not on anticoagulants or a known bleeder, then two common causes of an acute monarticular arthritis should be suspected: acute gout or a septic joint. Either one may be excruciatingly painful, but the grave danger lies in missing the diagnosis of a bacterial arthritis. A septic joint may be destroyed within forty-eight hours, hence rapid diagnosis and initiation of correct therapy are required.

The diagnostic procedure is a joint aspiration. It is quite easy to tap the knee medially under the patella if there is any effusion. Sterile technique should be used with care to avoid introducing bacteria into a previously sterile joint. The aspirate should be cultured, a sample should be placed in a heparinized tube to examine for crystals, a white blood cell count should be done with saline solution as a diluent, and a gram stain of a smear should be made. If the white cell count is attempted with the usual acetic acid diluent, the cells will clump in the precipitated mucus and the count will be falsely low. Someone experienced at looking for crystals should use a polarized light microscope to search for uric acid or the calcium pyrophosphate crystals seen in pseudogout. Cultures should be carefully done and should include an anaerobic culture using Thayer-Martin media for gonococcus. When evidence of gout or pseudogout is lacking, treatment for sepsis should be initiated without waiting for culture results if the joint leukocyte count is high.

A patient with a septic joint urgently needs hospitalization. Even if the correct diagnosis is gout, the patient deserves more rapid diagnosis and therapy than was given in this case. Most patients who come to the emergency room at 2 A.M. are in significant distress, and they deserve rapid, effective care.

On arrival at the rheumatology clinic two days after his emergency-room visit, this man's knee was tapped. The aspirated fluid had a white cell count of 15,500 per cu mm, and uric acid crystals were seen in some of the leukocytes. His acute attack was subsiding, and followup care was arranged.

Acute gout may be best treated acutely with colchicine (0.5 mg hourly by mouth) until the joint improves or diarrhea appears — they usually occur simultaneously — or with indomethacin (50 mg qid for one day and 25 mg qid for subsequent days) or with phenylbutazone (200 mg qid for one day and 100 mg qid thereafter). Before therapy is begun, the patient should have a CBC, blood uric acid, and rheumatoid preparation. The joint should be x-rayed, and followup should be arranged.

A 64-YEAR-OLD MAN was brought to the emergency room at
8 P.M. by his wife because of her concern that his scrotum was
swollen and tender. He was not too eager to obtain medical care
and volunteered little history but claimed to have been well previously and to have had scrotal swelling for about two days. He had
chilling but had not taken his temperature. He was not on any
medications and emphatically did not wish to remain in the hospital
as an inpatient.

On examination, the patient appeared slightly confused and ir-
ritable but in no other distress. His temperature was 38.8°C orally,
pulse 110, respiration 18, and blood pressure 150/90. His scrotum
was swollen, slightly edematous, tender throughout, and erythematous.
There was no remarkable inguinal lymphadenopathy. The scrotum
was so tender as to prevent careful palpation.

The patient was seen by a medical resident, who admitted that
the problem looked like some sort of an infection but that he had
never seen anything quite like it before. The man was also seen by
a urology resident, who admitted that he too had never seen such a
problem before. They elected to treat him with rest and oral antibiotics.

Two days later the patient had deteriorated further and was
brought back to the emergency room by his wife. He was more
obtunded and even less communicative than before. His scrotum
was further swollen and darker in color — almost black in areas —
and swelling extended up the thighs and lower abdomen. Slight
crepitus in the scrotum was noted.

This time the man was admitted to the hospital, and initial
laboratory studies indicated he was in diabetic ketoacidosis with a
high blood sugar level. Major surgical debridement of the scrotum
was done in the operating room. His subsequent hospital course
was very stormy, with an episode of acute renal failure.

What diseases predispose to bizarre infections?

What simple laboratory tests can be done in the emergency room to look for these predisposing disorders?

What organisms are most commonly responsible for gas gangrene?

Remarkable diseases should be remarked upon. This case puzzled both the medical and the urologic consultants, yet they were content to treat him as an example of a less bizarre illness and obtained no laboratory studies to search for other underlying diseases. They also did not pursue the problem of the patient's confusion.

Hematological disorders, diabetes mellitus, and uremia lead the list of diseases predisposing to unusual infections. A blood sugar, BUN, and CBC would have adequately screened for these and would have picked up the diabetes. Even a simple urinalysis would have allowed detection of the ketoacidosis. Missing this ancillary diagnosis surely allowed the infection to remain out of control despite antibiotic therapy.

Gas-forming bacteria are plentiful. The three most commonly seen are clostridia, bacteroids, and nonhemolytic streptococcus. Penicillin is usually the best antibiotic, but surgical drainage and debridement are essential, as is control of such associated problems as ketoacidosis. Ketoacidosis is itself a serious disorder with a significant mortality. It is usually viewed as a medical emergency requiring hospitalization and urgent therapy.

8

A 23-YEAR-OLD MAN was brought to the emergency room from the city jail one evening because he had become short-winded. He had suffered bronchial asthma since childhood and had been on corticosteroids in the past but not lately. His usual therapy consisted in oral Tedral tablets and an Isuprel inhaler. On the evening of his emergency-room admission, he had been arrested for verbally abusing a police officer who was trying to get him to move his car from an illegal parking area at an outdoor rock music festival. While in jail, the man had become short of breath and begun to wheeze. His jailers had him taken to the emergency room.

On arrival he appeared in only minimal respiratory distress. He was afebrile and had bilateral musical wheezes in his chest. An occasional nonproductive cough was apparent. His vital signs were: temperature 37.0°C, pulse 90, respiration 20, blood pressure 150/80.

Therapy was begun with oxygen by nasal prongs at a flow rate of 5 liters per minute, and an intravenous infusion of 500 mg of aminophylline in 500 ml of 5% dextrose solution was given over a two-hour period. At the end of this period the patient felt better, his wheezes were "less tight," and he was returned to the city jail.

During the next six hours he became dyspneic again and used his pocket isoproterenol (Isuprel) inhaler frequently in his jail cell. He was then returned to the emergency room, where he was seen almost immediately by a physician. His vital signs now were: temperature 37°C, pulse 110 and regular, respiration 22, blood pressure 154/82. His chest had diffuse wheezes but did seem to be ventilating adequately. He was not cyanotic. His heart sounded normal, and he had no edema. He was given 0.4 mg of epinephrine intramuscularly and within three minutes suffered a cardiac arrest. Despite vigorous immediate attempts at cardiopulmonary resuscitation, he could not be resuscitated.

Is epinephrine usually considered to be the drug of choice in treating asthma?

If this patient's death was not due purely to chance, what could have been the physiological state due to asthma prior to the epinephrine injection that predisposed him to a fatal arrhythmia?

What other disorders can present in the emergency room as "asthma"?

8 DISCUSSION

Asthma is a serious disease that is increasingly associated with sudden death, especially in users of inhaled bronchodilator aerosols. Asthmatics may become either alkalotic or acidotic. Either of these may be injurious, but in the setting of hypoxia and sympathomimetic loading, acidosis may be the more dangerous. Acidotic hypoxic hearts are very vulnerable to arrhythmias when sympathomimetics are given. If a sympathomimetic must be given when the patient might be hypoxic, it may be best not to give it by intravenous push or intramuscular or subcutaneous injection. The physician caring for the patient may not have fully appreciated the patient's self-administered "bronchodilator" and the possibility of serious hypoxia and pH abnormality. Infrequent premature ventricular contractions may have been present but missed.

Only an asthmatic given no prior therapy, with several hours of dyspnea at most, and with no notable fatigue now receives epinephrine in our emergency room. Pediatric asthma patients are somewhat different, and with them epinephrine may be less dangerous. Epinephrine is still usually considered the most effective drug in asthma, but in a patient already loaded with sympathomimetics the hazard of a fatal arrhythmia leads us to use other drugs.

Our recommended approach with an asthmatic is now as follows: give oxygen nasally and aminophylline plus fluids intravenously over one hour. At the end of that time, reevaluate the patient. If he is still dyspneic and not remarkably better, obtain an arterial blood-gas sample, a CBC, a chest x-ray, and a gram stain of any available sputum. If he has recently been on corticosteroids, give him a 300-mg bolus of hydrocortisone intravenously. If he has a fever, purulent-appearing sputum, or infiltrate on the chest x-ray, or fails to improve dramatically in four hours in the emergency room, he almost surely needs to be hospitalized. Fatigue is very dangerous and argues for admission.

Some asthmatics are regularly harder to treat than others. One may suspect that he is dealing with a difficult case when the patient relates that he has been on steroids in the past. Many very difficult cases of asthma are referred to special treatment centers, and a patient who has been so treated should be assumed to have asthma that does not respond easily to therapeutic efforts. The case described had such a history. Above all, the patient may be able to tell the doctor what therapy has been helpful or harmful to him in the past. Listen to him (of course, he may well ask for "a shot of Adrenalin"). Asthma is seldom easy to deal with.

The diagnosis of asthma is not always correct. Most commonly, the middle-aged or older patient who comes in claiming that his "asthma is giving him trouble" is *not* an asthmatic but rather has an exacerbation of chronic bronchitis, emphysema, or heart failure. As usual, the most important key to correct therapy is correct diagnosis, and one must not accept the patient's own diagnosis as correct. Obviously a patient in heart failure with "cardiac asthma" should not be given large amounts of fluids intravenously. A careful initial appraisal should seek evidence of heart failure such as elevated venous pressure or edema.

9

A 21-YEAR-OLD MAN came to the emergency room requesting a prescription for methadone. He stated that he was a heroin addict and used $30 to $50 worth of street heroin a day. He claimed heavy use of heroin for two years and heavy involvement in burglary to support his habit. Now he wished to stop taking the heroin and was feeling ill after having no drug for twelve hours.

On physical examination, no abnormalities were observed. The patient's veins were not scarred ("railroad tracks"); he had no round subcutaneous dimples (results of "skin popping"); and his pupils were midposition and reactive to light. Blood pressure was 130/50, pulse 95, respiration 16, and temperature 37.0°C.

The patient was given 40 mg of methadone (in 10-mg tablets) and left the emergency room. Six hours later he was returned to the emergency room deeply comatose but with adequate respiration and blood pressure. A friend stated that the patient had taken the methadone "to get high," that he had *not* been on heroin, and had drunk some vodka. His blood alcohol was 346 mg per 100 milliliters. Nalline, 5 mg given intravenously, produced no notable change, and the patient was kept in the emergency room under observation for twelve hours to "sleep it off."

What are the signs and symptoms of heroin withdrawal?

If a presumed heroin addict has seizures during a withdrawal period, what was he really taking?

Is methadone an innocuous drug?

This patient was obviously mainly drunk; however, the combination of methadone and alcohol is very dangerous, and the prescribing of methadone should be part of a maintenance program and not done in the emergency room. This patient was probably neither a heroin addict nor withdrawing from heroin.

Diaphoresis, dilated pupils, rhinorrhea, diarrhea, and colicky abdominal pain are early signs of narcotics withdrawal. Evidence of injection sites — usually needle tracks on arm veins — should be sought. People with inadequate veins (women, or chronic users in whom all available veins have thrombosed) may resort to "skin popping" or subcutaneous injection. They are prone to local abscesses and tetanus. (Thus, most cases of tetanus among narcotics addicts are in women.)

Seizures are not part of the narcotics withdrawal syndrome. Often street heroin or "horse" or "smack" is not truly heroin or contains only a small dose of heroin diluted with other drugs. Quinine, because it is white, powdery, and bitter, and produces flushing when given intravenously, is often mixed with barbiturate (for narcosis) unbeknown to the addict. Such a drug might lead to heroin withdrawal symptoms in an addict and later to barbiturate withdrawal symptoms such as seizures.

In general, it is best to treat a patient for narcotics withdrawal only when signs of that state are apparent and then to give 10 to 20 mg a day of methadone or other narcotic in equivalent dose while keeping the patient under observation. This dosage can be given until the patient is less ill or gets into a maintenance program. This dosage will take the edge off true heroin withdrawal symptoms but will not harm a user who is exaggerating his habit. It will not be enough to totally relieve an addict who is used to large doses of narcotics; he will still feel ill, even if not as ill as he would on no drug at all.

Methadone is widely used in the United States in maintenance therapy for chronic heroin addicts to prevent heroin euphoria and withdrawal symptoms. In such a program, a tolerant addict is usually given a daily dose of 60 to 120 mg of methadone. However, to a nontolerant person even 40 mg could be a very large dose. Mixed with alcohol or other sedatives, this amount of methadone can be fatal, acting as a respiratory depressant like any other narcotic.

A 24-YEAR-OLD MAN was brought to the emergency room and placed on an examining bed. He claimed to feel somewhat anxious and ill in an undefinable way and to need a shot of Thorazine. He denied using any drugs and refused to give any other history.

On examination his vital signs were as follows: blood pressure 160/90, pulse 110, respiration 18, temperature 37.4°C. His pupils were dilated, and he was very restless. He continually moved about the bed, making a 34- X 72-inch bed look like a football field by sitting in one corner then moving to another and then another. He had a fine tremor but no other neurologic signs. He appeared anxious and somewhat mistrustful, but was oriented to place, person, and time and had no obvious "hallucination lapses." He appeared normal through the rest of the examination. He continued to refuse to tell more about his problems.

Finally, after his requesting Thorazine over and over, the patient was given 25 mg of Thorazine intramuscularly, and he quickly calmed down. Later he admitted to having taken several amphetamine capsules a few hours before coming to the emergency room.

What is the differential diagnosis of a hyperanxious patient?

Do the dilated pupils help in the diagnosis?

What sorts of drug abuse can produce a hyperanxious state?

The hyperanxious patient may be suffering from a severe anxiety attack, may be evidencing symptoms of more severe underlying psychiatric illness, or may be suffering from a metabolic disorder. The metabolic disorders usually thought of in this syndrome include hypoglycemia, hyperthyroidism, pheochromocytoma, withdrawal from a sedative drug such as alcohol, and certain CNS drugs.

Evidence of sympathetic nervous system hyperactivity is present in most of these states, so slightly dilated pupils are not diagnostically helpful. However, widely dilated pupils argue for ingestion of certain drugs, especially those with strong parasympatholytic actions such as atropine or scopolamine.

The drugs we most often find incriminated as causes of acute panic include amphetamines, scopolamine (frequently present in over-the-counter sedative drugs), and hallucinogens. Amphetamines may render a person anxious, agitated, and possibly suicidal or homicidal. The patient often has a tachycardia and dilated pupils. Phenothiazines are very effective in this state, and most amphetamine users are aware of the effectiveness of Thorazine and other phenothiazines.

Amphetamines in usual doses seldom cause hallucinations. Although a drug abuser may not say that he is hallucinating, he may have pauses in his speech while he attends to the hallucination. Some hallucinating patients will politely excuse themselves for a few moments and then return their attention to the examiner. If the drug abuser is hallucinating, a very high dosage of amphetamines or other drugs, such as LSD, STP, or anticholinergics, should be suspected. Phenothiazines, which can cause hypotension in anyone, more easily produce hypotension in a patient on STP. Because of this, phenothiazines have been thought to be contraindicated with the hallucinogen. Even here, a small dose of Thorazine may be appropriate. In general, however, "talking the patient down" and small doses of diazepam (Valium) are preferable.

A drug abuser who is having a "bad trip" is often brought to the emergency room by friends who then quickly vanish to avoid "being busted" by any police officers who might be around. These friends may be the best source of information regarding the patient and his drugs, and they should be sought quickly when such a patient arrives.

Most drug users say that the "trip" depends not only on the drug itself but on circumstances and surroundings. A friendly, quiet atmosphere with friends present tends to produce a good trip, whereas a bad trip with frightening delusions and hallucinations will usually ensue if one ties the patient down on a hospital bed in a noisy, brightly lit cubicle. The emergency room is a very poor place to come down from an amphetamine high or a hallucinogen trip.

11

A 64-YEAR-OLD MAN was brought to the ER because of nosebleeds. His nose had been bleeding on and off for two days. He had placed some cotton in the left nostril for a few hours the day before his ER visit but then removed it. He was on no drugs, denied alcoholism, and had no known hypertension. There was no trauma to the nose, and family members who brought in the patient reported that he had been complaining of feeling tired that day.

The patient was placed on a bed with his head elevated. His blood pressure was 124/76 and pulse 70. He had a slow ooze of blood from his left nostril and sat clutching a blood-soaked terry-cloth towel. When he was stood up, he became dizzy and his blood pressure dropped to 70 systolic. No diastolic pressure was recorded. His pulse did not speed up noticeably on standing briefly. The inside of his left nostril was sprayed liberally with 4% cocaine, and then 4% cocaine was applied by cotton (twisted on a wire) into the nose. The left nostril was suctioned, but no precise bleeding point could be identified. A nasal pack with petroleum jelly—impregnated gauze was placed, and bleeding stopped. An intravenous infusion of normal saline solution was given through a large intracatheter in the patient's left arm; 2000 ml was given over one hour. Blood was sent for type and crossmatch (4 units were set up). The patient was admitted to the hospital for observation overnight.

How much blood is usually lost by epistaxis?

If bleeding stops after spraying phenylepherine (a vasoconstrictor) in the nose, should you pack the nose?

How long should the pack be left in place?

Epistaxis is probably the most common ear-nose-throat emergency. Although physicians usually underestimate blood loss when the blood is primarily external and visible, nonphysicians, especially patient's relatives, usually overestimate blood loss. Nonetheless, exsanguination via epistaxis can occur, and the physician should seek evidence of significant hypovolemia.

This patient's normal blood pressure was not known. Most 60-year-old men in this country have systolic blood pressures over 140, but 124 is not unusual and cannot be labeled low without a baseline value. One must use a stress test, such as sitting and then standing the patient: a young patient may preserve his blood pressure value but display a marked rise of pulse if hypovolemic. We consider a pulse rise of 35 beats per minute suggestive of a significant volume deficit. Older patients will often be unable to show an elevated pulse but may show a drop in blood pressure. Probably most important is the mean blood pressure, which can be estimated as diastolic BP plus one-third of pulse pressure. If the mean BP falls 15 mm Hg, the patient should be presumed to be significantly hypovolemic. A diastolic drop of more than 15 mm Hg is also often taken to indicate inadequate volume. If the patient shows an abnormal response to sitting, he should not be stood up.

Epistaxis does recur, and even if bleeding stops during the examination, the nose should be packed, at least on the offending side. The anterior nasal pack is usually adequate, and the doctor must pack with most pressure in the area that is bleeding. Nasal packing is painful, and anesthesia helps. A 4% cocaine spray or other local anesthetic can be used. The sphenopalatine ganglion may be injected by inserting a long needle through the foramen medial to the second molar (maxillary) just before the posterior edge of the hard palate. The nose goes back a long way, and it should be packed tightly and deeply. The nasal pack can be left in place for up to five days and removed in a followup visit to the ear-nose-throat clinic. We often prescribe an antibiotic such as ampi-cillin, 250 mg orally qid, while the pack is in place.

12

A 34-YEAR-OLD WOMAN walked into the emergency room accompanied by her aunt. The patient was obviously very frightened, and tears were running down her face, but she spoke with very little movement of her mouth and claimed that she had "lockjaw." The aunt furnished the following information: the patient had been well until one week earlier, when she had had some cramping low abdominal pain and nausea. She had seen her physician, who had given her some yellow capsules. The pain and nausea had lessened, but for the past two days she had had trouble using her mouth, and today it had "locked on her." She recalled no trauma or puncture wounds and denied any experimental use of drugs, "pill popping," or "shooting up" of drugs. The yellow pills were unavailable.

On examination the vital signs were observed as follows: temperature 37.0°C, pulse 100, blood pressure 140/85, respiration 18. The patient's chest and heart were normal, and deep tendon reflexes were normal. Her gait was unremarkable, and muscle tone seemed normal. Her jaw was tightly clenched, but on coaxing she could open it for examination. No pharyngeal, ear, or neck pathology could be found.

One of the examining physicians at first felt the patient had a paratonsillar abscess or, failing that, a hysterical conversion reaction. To add to the confusion, the woman's aunt was loudly chanting prayers for her relief. Fortunately, an alert nurse correctly diagnosed the problem. The patient was given an intravenous injection and immediately remarked that she felt better. Within five minutes the jaw tightness was entirely gone. The patient left for home within thirty minutes of her arrival in the emergency room.

What was the matter with this woman?

What was in the yellow capsules?

What drug was given to her in the ER?

12 DISCUSSION

The patient exemplifies an acute onset of an extrapyramidal movement disorder. These are usually due to phenothiazines and are essentially unrelated to the dose, being an idiosyncratic reaction. The differential diagnosis must include: (1) tetanus, (2) strychnine (now uncommon as a primary ingestant but not infrequently combined with hallucinogens such as STP, DME, or LSD), and (3) hysteria. Indeed, the unsophisticated physician usually picks hysteria as an explanation for phenothiazine reactions, and at one time almost all extrapyramidal diseases were thought to be hysterical since the movements are exacerbated by anxiety and improved by tranquillity.

These movement disorders can present as dystonias such as torticollis, oculogyric crisis (the patient may complain that he can't get his eyes off the ceiling), or total body writhing. The patient may have spasmodic movements with leg-jerking, head-bobbing, or choreiform total body hyperactivity (akathisia). Localized muscle tone increases may vary from this patient's sense of jaw tightness or tongue protrusion to opisthotonos and extensor rigidity throughout the body.

This patient had been on an antiemetic and "GI antispasmodic" marketed as Combid. Probably any phenothiazine can lead to movement disorders, and the frequency with which they do so is proportional to the frequency with which physicians prescribe them. There are several effective therapies. The offending drug must be stopped. If the movement disorder is of recent onset, diphenhydramine (Benadryl) given orally or intravenously will rapidly reduce symptoms. We usually give 50 mg intravenously to produce a dramatic improvement that is very reassuring to the patient. Then we continue the patient on 50 mg orally qid for several days. This was the therapy used on the patient described.

13

A 45-YEAR-OLD MAN was found in his room after neighbors heard a gunshot. The door was forced and he was found in a pool of blood with a small-caliber revolver in his hand. It appeared that he had pointed the gun in his mouth and fired. An ambulance was called, and it responded promptly, with a total time from initial call to arrival at the emergency room of eleven minutes. On arrival, the patient was unconscious; there was no palpable pulse or audible heartbeat; no respiratory movements were present; his pupils were fixed and dilated; his mouth was full of blood.

Initial resuscitative efforts were directed to establishing an airway. The mouth was suctioned, and an endotracheal tube was placed orally. Ventilation could not be established. Later closer examination showed that the endotracheal tube had entered not the trachea but rather the bullet tract in the posterior pharynx. After the patient had been declared dead, a lateral skull and neck x-ray view showed the presence of an air pneumogram.

How else might an airway have been established in a patient with such an oral injury?

How can one determine whether a patient is a candidate for a resuscitative effort rather than being declared DOA (dead on arrival)?

13 DISCUSSION

First-aid measures begin with establishing an airway. Other primary first-aid goals include stopping bleeding, treating shock, sealing sucking chest wounds, and preventing further trauma by splinting. Resuscitative measures must also begin with these same goals. In most well-equipped, well-staffed emergency rooms the favorite method of airway establishment is oral endotracheal intubation. This is most easily done with a curved laryngoscope blade inserted anteriorly to the epiglottis so as to lift the entire larynx, with the patient supine, with head forward in the "sniffing position," and with a stylet in the endotracheal tube for good control.

Oral intubation is difficult or impossible in several situations. A patient may present with clenched teeth even with rather deep coma. Oral intubation must be preceded by muscle paralysis (e.g., with succinyl choline) in such a case, or nasal tracheal intubation or cricothyroidotomy must be used. A patient who is too conscious to tolerate oral intubation may well tolerate nasal tracheal intubation. A patient with extensive mouth or jaw damage or bleeding or with obstruction to the vocal cords due to foreign objects, emesis, or bleeding can best have an airway established by cricothyroidotomy. The cricothyroid membrane is palpable directly beneath the skin between the thyroid cartilage ("Adam's apple") and the cricoid cartilage. A transverse incision can go through skin and membrane and be immediately followed by insertion of a finger or other dilating instrument, such as a surgical clamp, and then an endotracheal tube. Although such an airway lacks many of the advantages of a conventional tracheostomy, it can be maintained for over twenty-four hours without serious increased risk of bad sequelae. This is the procedure usually referred to as an "emergency tracheostomy." It is the procedure performed with penknives to rescue persons with "café coronaries" (acute upper airway obstruction by a large foreign body — usually unchewed steak in an intoxicated restaurant patron). A standard tracheostomy is at least a ten-minute procedure by good surgeons in the best of circumstances and has no place in establishing an emergency airway.

The decision to attempt to resuscitate someone who has apparently died should logically take into consideration the patient's primary disease or diseases, the time the patient has been anoxic, the temperature of the body (the brain can tolerate hypoxia longer if it has been chilled than it can at 37.0°C), and the patient's age. However, at the time, little of this information is usually available, and the only true test of resuscitability of a patient is the success or failure of an adequate attempt at resuscitation by a skilled crew with adequate equipment. Although such a resuscitation may be successful only to the extent of producing a "vegetable" who needs constant mechanical ventilation, is in coma, and has a viable heartbeat only until pneumonia finally brings death, nonetheless the decision of the resuscitation team must be to go ahead with the resuscitation attempt. A later decision to discontinue artificial ventilation and other life support mechanisms may be necessary, but the initial decision should be to attempt resuscitation.

Dilated pupils that are "fixed" (unresponsive to light) are often cited as incontrovertible evidence of death or nonresuscitability. This is incorrect. Especially in young persons or persons who have taken drug overdoses, fixed, dilated pupils may be present with later total recovery of the patient.

14

A 29-YEAR-OLD WOMAN came to the emergency room complaining of "hyperventilating." She had suffered for years from chronic anxiety and had previously had many anxiety attacks accompanied by rapid breathing and weakness. Sometimes she would have paresthesias, and she had learned to treat the attacks by breathing in a paper bag. Aside from a regular alcohol consumption of several drinks daily, she had no other known medical problems.

On the day before her emergency-room visit, as she was driving home from the divorce court — where she had just obtained a final divorce decree — she noted the onset of rapid breathing with a sense of dyspnea and within minutes noted the onset of a pounding, rapid heartbeat in her chest. She felt weak but continued driving home. Bag breathing gave her no relief. None of her previous episodes of hyperventilation had been accompanied by palpitations. Eighteen hours later, at 4 A.M., she became worried enough about the palpitations, dyspnea, tachypnea, and weakness to call for an ambulance to bring her to the emergency room.

On arrival the patient was anxious and in some evident distress. She was afebrile and showed acrocyanosis with cool extremities. She had a deep rapid respiration (a rate of 35), tachycardia (cardiac rate 160 and regular), and blood pressure of 150/85. Her jugular venous pressure seemed normal. She had a clear chest, unremarkable heart sounds, and no edema. A brief neurologic exam showed no abnormality. She had no facial twitching on tapping the facial nerve just anterior to the ear (Chvostek sign) and no carpal spasm on placing a BP cuff around the upper arm and holding it at 170 mm Hg for three minutes (Trousseau sign).

An electrocardiogram showed a regular supraventricular tachycardia that the physician present felt was paroxysmal atrial tachycardia (PAT). Carotid massage and gagging maneuvers produced no change. An intravenous route was established, and the patient was given Digoxin, 0.5 mg intravenously. Neither this nor subsequent carotid massage nor a further 0.5 mg of Digoxin led to any change. An arterial blood-gas sample was obtained and showed a pH of 7.08, pCO_2 18, and pO_2 110. The acidosis was noted and thought probably to be a lactic acidosis resulting from tissue hypoperfusion due to the tachycardia. Physostigmine (2 mg) was given intravenously, followed by ampules of $NaHCO_3$ (44 mEq each), with no change in her condition. Edrophonium (Tensilon) (10 mg) was given intravenously, and the patient's cardiac rate slowed from 160 to 130. This was felt to be remarkable — since PAT always converts abruptly or does not change at all — and redirected attention to her acidosis. She denied ingesting methanol, antifreeze, or aspirin. A urinalysis was done and showed glucose (4 +) and a large amount of acetone. She was admitted to the ward with the diagnosis of diabetic keto-acidosis in a previously undiagnosed diabetic. Later she recalled that her mother had adult-onset diabetes.

What possibilities did the arterial blood gas levels reveal?

Is there any danger in bicarbonate therapy of the acidosis?

What is the danger of digitalis in an acidotic patient?

Hyperventilation is too often identified as a psychological problem, whereas it frequently is caused by serious lung disease or a metabolic acidosis. A normal pCO_2 at sea level is about 40 mm Hg. At Denver (elevation 5280 feet, barometric pressure 630 mm Hg) a slight hyperventilation produces a slight decrease of the pCO_2 to about 37 mm Hg. This patient showed a marked decrease of the pCO_2, thus might have been expected to show an alkalosis. Since the patient was not only not alkalotic but was severely acidotic, she had a metabolic acidosis.

There are four main causes of metabolic acidosis. The most common in a young person is diabetic ketoacidosis, and the cardinal error in this case seemed to be neglecting to do a urinalysis when presented with a hyperventilating patient. If a urine specimen had been examined, the diagnosis would have been apparent before costly time was wasted and potentially dangerous maneuvers undertaken. Less common causes of metabolic acidosis are exogenous poisons (especially methanol and salicylate), renal disease with uremia or renal tubular acidosis, and lactic acidosis (usually with gross tissue hypoxia and often due to shock).

Treatment of metabolic acidosis with $NaHCO_3$ is reasonable and can lessen the risk of fatal cardiac arrhythmias. However, the HCO_3 is denied easy access to the cerebrospinal fluid, and the brief increase of pCO_2 by the reaction

$$H^+ + HCO_3^- \rightleftharpoons H_2CO_3 \rightleftharpoons H_2O + CO_2$$

will allow for an increased CSF pCO_2 and a paradoxical increase in H^+ concentration in the CSF — thus a decrease in CSF pH. This may produce coma or seizures.

Digitalis is a dangerous drug. It can produce serious arrhythmias, especially if given in a setting of hypoxia or acidosis. Although probably the first choice drug in treating a patient with PAT, further use of digitalis in a setting of sinus tachycardia and acidosis can only be hazardous and not helpful.

Perhaps the moral of this story is that, given time, a good doctor will eventually find his way to the correct diagnosis. If he hasn't done too much harm along the way, the patient will eventually benefit from his attentions.

15

A 30-YEAR-OLD WOMAN was in the back of a camper truck when it was involved in an accident. There was a momentary gas explosion that produced a flash of flame but no subsequent fire. The woman was brought to the emergency room by ambulance. When she arrived, she was complaining of painful hands and legs. She had blistering burns over most of her legs and her hands but seemed otherwise unharmed. Her face was unhurt, and there was no charring or reddening of her mouth. Her vital signs were normal, and she was breathing easily with a rate of sixteen.

What requires first evaluation in a burned patient?

How would you treat this patient in the ER?

What pulmonary problem could develop in the ensuing twenty-four hours?

The state of the airway is our first concern in a burn case, just as it is in all major emergencies. If the mouth seems reddened or charred, or there is much evidence of facial burning, or the patient is dyspneic or has stridor, we pass an endotracheal tube and later do a tracheostomy. In this case the airway did not seem endangered.

We first establish two large intravenous portals, one of which must serve as a central venous pressure manometer. We then give narcotics intravenously for analgesia and wrap much of the burned areas with towels soaked in iced saline solution. This provides some analgesia and cleansing. Often the patient is then taken to the operating room for careful debridement under general anesthesia and for dressing with an antibacterial agent such as silver nitrate.

If there was a significant amount of smoke present and inhaled, a chemical pneumonitis or pulmonary edema could develop in the next day or two. This can produce serious hypoxia and may require placing the patient on a ventilator. In this case there was little smoke, and there were no late respiratory sequelae.

16

A 26-YEAR-OLD MAN parked his car and walked into the emergency room. He complained of headache, dizziness, nausea, and tiredness. He commented that he had just finished a 180-mile drive over snow-drifted mountain highways at an average speed of 20 mph and that his car had been leaking fumes continuously. He thought he was suffering from carbon monoxide poisoning.

On physical examination the patient was alert and in no apparent distress. His vital signs were normal except for a blood pressure of 160/100, and he had some mild ataxia. His skin was a bright pink color. Otherwise, he appeared to be normal.

How can his diagnosis be documented?

If arterial blood gas analyses were done, what might they show?

What should his therapy be?

This indeed sounds like carbon monoxide poisoning. Many patients with this disorder who are conscious on arrival at the emergency room are able to make their own diagnoses. The usual symptoms include headache, nausea and vomiting, loss of consciousness, and extra-pyramidal disorders such as posturing, dystonic movements, tremor, and ataxia. The physical exam is usually said to show a "cherry red skin," but this is more often a pink color. Dyspnea is not prominent, nor is tachypnea.

A blood sample can be drawn for carboxyhemoglobin. In this case the reading was 38%; thus, 38% of the patient's hemoglobin was bound by carbon monoxide. This would seem to mean that 62% of the hemoglobin is available for O_2 binding — a situation similar to that in anemia, where about one-third of the red cell mass is lost. However, the carboxyhemoglobin also produces a shift of the hemoglobin dissociation curve to the left, producing a greater saturation for a given oxygen tension. The point here is that the tissue oxygen tensions must be very low for the hemoglobin to unload its oxygen to the tissue fluid. This makes the situation even worse for the patient.

An arterial blood gas determination in a case such as this would show a normal pO_2 as long as ventilation is adequate and a seemingly normal O_2 saturation since this is determined colorimetrically and carboxyhemoglobin falsely reads as oxyhemoglobin.

Therapy should be primarily high-flow oxygen. If the patient is unconscious, coma precautions should be taken. He should be lying in a lateral decubitus position, with his mouth down and off the bed to avoid aspiration in the event of vomiting. An endotracheal tube should be placed, since the patient's airway is in danger, and his ventilation assisted with 100% O_2.

This patient was treated simply with nasal oxygen at 15 liters per minute. He was given a paper bag to hold over his nose and mouth to act as an oxygen reservoir. Within two hours his headache was gone, his pink skin color had faded, and he was no longer ataxic. He was discharged to go home within four hours of arrival in the ER. Late cerebral complications with coma have occurred in carbon

monoxide poisoning but are rare if the patient was not comatose
originally.

A 65-YEAR-OLD MAN was brought to the emergency room by ambulance. He had passed out on a downtown sidewalk, and the ambulance was called by bystanders. On arrival, the patient insisted that he felt well. He claimed to be a "fainter." He had fainted over fifteen times in the last year. During these faints, which lasted no more than a few minutes, he was never incontinent and had no remarkable movements. There was no aura or warning, but he had never hurt himself in a fall. The man was visiting from another city, where he was under the care of a Veterans Administration hospital cardiologist for these faints. He was planning to return home the very next day and in fact had an appointment with his physician within a week. He denied any other symptoms and was on no medications.

The physical examination revealed nothing remarkable. Blood pressure was 140/80, pulse 80 and regular, respiratory rate 15, temperature 37.0°C, and jugular venous pressure seemed within normal limits. The patient was alert, well-oriented, and had no gross neurologic defects. An electrocardiogram showed right bundle branch block (RBBB) and first-degree atrioventricular (AV) block with a PR interval of 0.26 seconds.

The patient wanted no therapy and minimized the event. He was discharged to return to the care of his physician in his home city. Twelve hours later he was brought back to the emergency room, having expired suddenly. He was dead on arrival, and no resuscitation was attempted.

What is the significance of coexistent RBB block and first-degree AV block?

What other ECG abnormalities might have the same ominous portent?

What might best have been done for the patient when he came to the ER?

The history and setting are classic for Adams-Stokes attacks: loss of consciousness that follows the development of complete heart block with attendant ventricular fibrillation, ventricular tachycardia, or asystole. The heart block and attendant arrhythmia may be intermittent, and the patient may die during an attack, as probably happened in this case.

Not all cardiac causes of syncope are signaled by the electrocardiogram. However, some ECG signs are important as probable progenitors of complete heart block and consequently the liability of sudden death. These are right bundle branch block (RBBB) with left axis deviation (LAD) of the unblocked early (QRS) forces, Mobitz type-II block (complete sudden failure for a beat to conduct), alternating right and left bundle branch block, LBBB masquerading as RBBB, and some instances of either RBBB or LBBB with first-degree AV block. These ECG patterns reflect bilateral bundle branch disease. It may be a small step from such bilateral disease to complete heart block, and the history of syncope bridges this gap.

In rare instances the ECG will make the diagnosis of a myocardial infarction that was silent except for the syncope. Occasionally myocardial defects or valvular lesions associated with loss of consciousness, such as aortic stenosis, may be found through patient history, physical examination, or ECG.

With a resting ECG abnormality suggestive of periods of severe AV block and with a history of many faints, this patient should probably have had a demand pacemaker inserted. One probably should assume that any fainter might die with the next faint, and a pacemaker could be counted on to take over if the patient's own conduction system failed. The fact that he had not died with previous faints does not make further episodes of AV block less dangerous. The actual mechanism of death in this patient was not determined, but it seems most likely to have been a blockage of atrioventricular conduction.

Syncope is a common presenting problem in most emergency rooms. Most patients have no suggestions of a seizure in their histories, and few have helpful electrocardiograms. Perhaps more patients should be admitted to hospitals for monitoring purposes even with normal electrocardiograms.

A 22-YEAR-OLD WOMAN came to the emergency room because she had been suffering with chest pain for four days and was getting no better. She had been well until two weeks earlier, when she developed a "cold": rhinorrhea, sore throat, and a dry cough. She had taken no medications other than her usual oral contraceptives and was no worse until she suddenly had right lateral chest pain on arising one morning. The pain was aggravated by movement and by coughing. She had no chills, did not take her temperature, and did not produce sputum. She was allergic to no medications, had had no contact with birds or other animals, had no past tuberculosis contacts, and, although plump, usually enjoyed excellent health.

The patient's vital signs were normal. Chest sounds were dull at the right base, and there were decreased breath sounds at the right base. She was in some distress from chest pain on movement. She had no leg tenderness and no edema. Her cardiac examination showed nothing abnormal, and her second sound seemed normal.

A chest x-ray showed an effusion in the right pleural space and a small infiltrate in the right lower lung field, interpreted as probably a viral pneumonia by the radiologist.

What is the diagnostic problem here?

Is the patient in any significant danger?

What would you do for this patient?

18 DISCUSSION

The diagnostic problem here is largely distinguishing between a pulmonary embolism with infarction and a pneumonia with effusion. If embolism is the correct diagnosis, the danger is that another, larger embolus may be forthcoming and may prove fatal. The problem is usually not *this* embolus but the next one.

An arterial blood gas analysis may show hypoxemia (in Denver, pO_2 below 65 mm Hg) with normal or low pCO_2 in either disease state. A normal arterial blood sample might be found at this time, four days into her history. A lung scan could be done and would be helpful if it shows filling defects in areas normal on the chest x-ray. It will probably show the defect seen on the x-ray in either disorder. If the scan shows other defects, pulmonary emboli are probable.

The absence of peripheral venous obstruction signs or symptoms is in no way a significant argument against the diagnosis of pulmonary embolism and infarction. Venous findings are present in less than half the cases of documented pulmonary emboli. The most helpful cardiac finding arguing for pulmonary embolism is an increased volume of the second component of the second heart sound in the pulmonic area.

The major therapeutic dilemma is whether or not to give the patient an anticoagulant. To make this decision one really needs a pulmonary angiogram in most cases. Probably the best approach in this case would be to admit the patient to the hospital for angiography and possibly heparinization. All too often such a patient has less diagnostic procedures done with equivocal results, is sent home on antibiotics, and suffers a recurrence of pulmonary embolism. At this late date, even angiography might not be helpful, and a decision to place the patient on anticoagulants might have to be made without clear-cut evidence of embolic disease.

19

A 30-YEAR-OLD MAN, a psychologist, came to the emergency room complaining of severe left-sided throbbing headaches over the preceding two weeks. The headaches involved the left face from brow to maxilla and centered about the left eye. During headaches which lasted for several hours he often vomited, and this seemed to relieve the pain somewhat. He had no family history of headache, no juvenile carsickness or frequent nausea, and recalled no head trauma. He noted that one of his more severe episodes had followed an alcoholic drink, but usually he did not drink or smoke. Although one headache had awakened him, the rest had been during the daytime hours. About three years earlier he had suffered several similar headaches over a two-month period. He was on no drugs except aspirin, which gave him little relief.

On physical examination he appeared to be a normal man in no apparent distress. Vital signs were normal: temperature 37.0°C and blood pressure 130/80. His pain was now gone, and his conjunctivas were normal, although he thought the left eye was sometimes bloodshot with the pain. There were no audible bruits over the skull and no tenderness over the sinuses, and fundi and tympanic membranes were normal. The neck was supple, and the patient appeared entirely normal on a careful neurologic exam and a brief general physical exam.

What should be examined when a patient complains of headache?

What sort of headache syndromes are most common in the ER?

When does a patient deserve a spinal tap?

What is the diagnosis in this case?

19 DISCUSSION

The patient history information needed to evaluate a case of headache includes the following: Where is the headache? Is it unilateral or bilateral? Does it pound with the pulse, or is it a steady headache? (It is important to avoid using the word "only" in discussing this matter with the patient, as in "Is your headache pounding or *only* steady?") Does the patient have a fever or chills? Has he been suffering from upper respiratory symptoms such as runny nose, stuffy head, earache, ringing in ears, sore throat, or hoarseness? Was there any previous head trauma? Has he been having blurred or double vision, nausea, or vomiting? Has he had high blood pressure in the past? What drugs is he taking and what is he allergic to? Does coughing or sneezing exacerbate the headache? Is there photophobia? How does he try to relieve the pain? Are there any warnings before the headache?

The physical findings that it is important to elicit in any case of headache include the following: Check for tenderness of the skull and the maxillary and frontal sinuses. The frontal sinuses must be felt from under the supraorbital ridge as opposed to the maxillary sinuses, which can be palpated directly. Check the equality of the pupils and their response to light. Evaluate the presence of nystagmus. Take temperature, pulse, respiration, and blood pressure. Check flexibility of the neck with the patient attempting to put his ears on his shoulders and to flex his chin on his chest. Observe his gait and his deep tendon reflexes. Examine the optic fundi for papilledema or hemorrhages.

Headache syndromes which present in the emergency room usually include the following:

1. Febrile headaches — usually bilateral and present with a fever of at least 38.4°C. This headache may be steady but is often pounding. Of course, the source of the fever must be found, and this may turn out to be as simple as a urinary tract infection, respiratory tract infection, or viral flu syndrome.
2. Muscular headache — usually bilateral and mainly in the back of the head. It is steady and worse in the evening. It may

last for days. It is the most common headache syndrome
seen and usually responds to salicylates or other mild pain
medications, such as Darvon.
3. Vascular headaches — usually classified as (a) atypical or common migraine or (b) typical or uncommon migraine. The point of
this is that the vascular headache usually seen does not have
all the features of classic migraine. The classic migraine headache is a unilateral, pounding headache with visual changes,
nausea, and vomiting; it lasts for hours, and there is a strong
family history of headaches. However, the more common
varieties often lack some of these features and may have no
prodrome. In addition, a vascular headache often eventually
develops into a muscular headache. If caught early enough,
a vascular headache can be treated with ergot. In the emergency
room, this can be ergotamine tartrate in an injectable form.
Once the headache has progressed, though, the best treatment
is usually strong analgesics, especially narcotics. We usually
give a dose of meperadine or morphine or codeine and try to
get the patient home.
4. Sinus headaches — extremely rare. Most patients who come
in complaining of sinus headaches are actually complaining
of other sorts of headaches. If the patient indeed has a fever
and is tender over the sinuses, a set of sinus films should be
obtained and a throat culture should be taken. In adults,
usually sinus headaches are caused by streptococcal infections
or viral infections. Treatment should, of course, include antibiotics if the physician suspects that streptococcus is present,
and the antibiotic of choice is penicillin. The more important
features of the treatment are analgesics and decongestants.
5. Hypertension headache — generally in the back of the head
and often worse in the morning. The diastolic blood pressure
should be at least 110 mm Hg to make this diagnosis. The
problem is increased by the fact that many people get a
temporary elevation of the diastolic blood pressure with pain
anywhere, including headache.
6. Post head-trauma headache — usually involves all of the head.
Patients who have been hit on the head (especially if they

have suffered concussion) have a syndrome consisting of headache, light-headedness, and malaise which may last for weeks or even months. Dizziness is usually severe on rapid standing and is increased by almost any treatment we might use for the headaches, other than salicylates. The patient's affect may be depressed, and he may find himself neurotic and unable to do his usual work. Some people have used terms such as "organic neurosis" for this syndrome. The most important part of the therapy is to reassure the patient. The patient should be told that his syndrome occurs following head trauma, that it always goes away within weeks or months, and that the least treatment is the best treatment.

7. Although eye problems are often suggested, they are very rare as a cause of headache. However, glaucoma should be kept in mind.

8. Dental problems also can cause headaches in rare instances, but one should consider trigeminal neuralgia or temporal mandibular joint arthritis.

Any headache patient who has remarkable physical findings and who does not seem to fit clearly in any of the above categories may have more serious organic brain disease. The physical examination recommended here for headache workup is actually quite brief and can be done in about four minutes. Remarkable findings will be made in only about 3% or fewer of the patients arriving at the emergency room with complaints of headache. These patients may need further workup for disorders such as brain tumor and other intracranial pathology. Patients making repeated visits for severe headache usually deserve a spinal tap to rule out chronic meningitis. The adage "When you think of it, do it" holds most of the time for a spinal tap. A patient who says that his present headache is *the worst he has ever had* probably deserves a tap to rule out meningitis (a treatable cause of severe acute headache) or a subarachnoid hemorrhage.

In this case the patient probably had a vascular headache known as cluster migraine or Horton's histamine cephalalgia. Therapy with Cafergot (ergotamine plus caffeine) aborted many of his subsequent headaches, but he still eventually needed therapy with methysergide (Sansert).

20

A 21-YEAR-OLD WOMAN came to the emergency room complaining of recent contact with gonorrhea. She said she felt well but her boyfriend had just called her to say that he had a gonococcal infection. She had been having sexual intercourse with him frequently. The doctor who saw her recommended that she return if she began to show symptoms.

Would there be any benefit from a pelvic examination in this case?

What culture techniques are used for gonorrhea?

If you decided that the patient had the disease, what therapy would you give her?

What are the likely consequences of the approach used in this case?

Most women with gonococcal cervicitis show no symptoms, perhaps for months or years. Nonetheless, if therapy is withheld, the patient may well go on to develop acute pelvic inflammatory disease or distant septic spread, such as gonococcal arthritis.

The patient should be examined. The cervical os should be cultured after an initial swabbing to remove as much cervical mucus as possible. A culture should be done on warm Thayer-Martin medium. The next most useful sites for culture are the anal canal and the urethra, in that order. A gram stain of the cervix is not very helpful, for it is often negative when cultures are positive and sometimes falsely read as positive due to the presence of pleomorphic gram-negative rods.

Our present recommended therapy for gonorrhea in a man or woman who is not allergic to penicillin is procaine penicillin G, 4.8 million units intramuscularly, plus 1 gm of probenecid given in one dose. In a penicillin-sensitive patient we usually use Vibramycin, 200 mg daily for five days, or spectinomycin. The most common complication of untreated or inadequately treated gonorrhea in a woman will be a persistent subclinical infection. She will be able to transmit this infection to her boyfriend after he is cured or to any other male contacts.

If not treated, the patient may well become acutely ill, with nausea and vomiting, lower abdominal pain and tenderness, fever and leukocytosis, and rebound tenderness with peritonitis, all of which make differentiation from appendicitis difficult. This acute pelvic inflammatory disease may require hospitalization with parenteral high-dose antibiotics therapy and may render her sterile thereafter. Such an acute illness may develop weeks or months after her initial contact with gonorrhea.

Early treatment of asymptomatic gonorrhea is essential and would be recommended in this case. In fact, therapy without a pelvic examination would have been acceptable even if not optimal. Lack of therapy was unacceptable. We automatically treat known female contacts of men who have gonorrhea. We do not wait for the results of the culture to begin therapy when there is a suggestive history as in this case.

21

A 36-YEAR-OLD MAN was brought to the emergency room by a concerned friend who promptly vanished. The patient claimed that he was "going into the DTs." He had been drinking heavily for about sixteen years and had been dry for no more than four months at a time during that period. His present binge had lasted three weeks. He had been drinking mainly vodka at a rate of over a fifth a day, but the past few days he had been drinking wine, and today his money had run out. His last drink had been six hours before he came to the ER. Between binges he had worked as a laborer, dishwasher, and cook. He smoked two packs of cigarettes a day and denied a cough except for "a smoker's cough." During the preceding few days he had been nauseated and had vomited several times, especially in the mornings. The vomiting did not follow a coughing spell, and after taking a drink ("the hair of the dog that bit him") he felt better. Now he felt shaky, nauseated, and generally very sick. He claimed to be hallucinating when left alone: "seeing animals on the wall." He said he "needed a drink badly" and asked for an injection of Librium.

On physical examination the patient was tremulous and anxious, and looked ill. He was wasted and unshaven. His right hand had multiple nicotine stains. His clothes smelled of urine and other, unidentifiable odors. Vital signs included blood pressure 160/110 in the right arm when recumbent, 140/100 standing, pulse 130, respiratory rate 25, temperature 38.1°C. His venous pressure seemed normal. His eyes were bloodshot; his chest had audible bilateral coarse wheezes; his abdomen was diffusely moderately tender; and his legs and feet seemed inordinately sensitive to stroking or pressure. He would jerk his leg away when the sole of the foot was touched.

Why do alcoholics stop drinking?

Does this patient have delirium tremens?

Can alcohol withdrawal symptoms appear within six hours of
the last drink?

The *binge drinker* can be dry for months but is drunk for days or weeks when he drinks. His binge is generally ended in one of three ways. He may be arrested by the police for "being drunk in a public place" or "driving while under the influence of alcohol" (DUI), and once in jail he will begin to suffer withdrawal symptoms. He may suffer an attack of acute gastritis, pancreatitis, or pneumonia that will render him too ill to continue to drink. Most commonly, he will run out of money. In this setting he may taper off over several days with wine or beer.

The earliest withdrawal symptoms are usually nausea and vomiting, notably the morning after a binge. These are treatable with alcohol and so represent withdrawal symptoms rather than gastritis or other intra-abdominal pathology. Then tremor, anxiety, and malaise become prominent. Many withdrawing alcoholics seem unable to define their symptoms beyond being "sick."

Fever is common, as is tachycardia, in alcohol withdrawal. However, almost all drinkers are heavy smokers. The alcohol suppresses the white blood cell count (folate deficiency and direct bone marrow suppression) and the pulmonary muco-ciliary apparatus. The cigarette smoke is a chronic irritant, making the patient prone to bronchitis, pneumonia, and tuberculosis. Gastrointestinal bleeding is common in alcoholics. Such a patient should have pulse and blood pressure taken supine and upright to look for evidence of hypovolemia. He also must have a rectal examination and a stool test for occult blood.

Head trauma is common in alcoholics, and chronic or acute subdural hematomas are prevalent. Confusion and ataxia should not be accepted too quickly as due to alcohol intoxication (a blood alcohol will help here) or withdrawal.

Hallucinations — deranged and distorted sensory perceptions — are common in alcohol withdrawal. They may begin as nightmares, then go on to include hallucinations when the patient is alone in a dark room. Next there may be visual (seldom auditory) hallucinations even in well-lighted rooms. All these are generally ego-alien to the patient: He recognizes them as frightening but unreal. Only after many days are the hallucinations ego-syntonic and the patient truly lost within them.

Delirium tremens (DTs) is a rare syndrome in a withdrawing alcoholic who does not also have an associated illness such as pancreatitis or some major trauma (accidentally or surgically incurred). The DT patient is totally disoriented, agitated, and unable to remove himself from his hallucinations. He has a tachycardia and often a very high fever. He does *not* arrive able to tell us that he is "going into DTs." And delirium tremens requires intensive care.

This patient seems to have an alcohol withdrawal syndrome with tremor, nausea and vomiting, tachycardia, and focal hallucinations. He also has chronic bronchitis. The alcohol withdrawal syndrome may develop even while the person is still drinking as long as his intake and blood alcohol level are dropping. One should not assume this patient's blood alcohol to be zero — he may have had several drinks more recently than he tells us.

22

A 36-YEAR-OLD MAN was seen in another emergency room following an auto accident. He was thought to have a fractured humerus.
His blood pressure was noted to be 90/50, and an intravenous infusion was begun with 5% dextrose in water through a 25-gauge
scalp vein needle. He was given 16 mg of morphine sulfate for pain
and was transferred by ambulance to the Denver General Hospital
emergency room with a diagnosis of "mild shock." On arrival he
had a blood pressure of 70/40, clammy skin, and a pulse rate of 140.
Three large intravenous routes were introduced with short 16-gauge
intracatheters, and 4 liters of saline solution were given over one
hour. Blood pressure rose to 110/60 and remained stable. The
patient's abdomen was tender, and x-rays showed he had several
fractured ribs and a fractured humerus. At laparotomy soon after,
the surgeon removed a fractured spleen.

What constitutes an emergency?

How do you recognize that an emergency is present?

Is "mild shock" similar to "slightly pregnant"?

Should one use a long CVP catheter from the right anticubital
fossa to the superior vena cava in acutely traumatized patients?

There are not really many cases that demand urgent care in the first thirty minutes. Most of these can be identified by attention to the patient's chief complaint, mental status, and vital signs. True emergencies present as problems in the central nervous system, the respiratory system, or the cardiovascular system. Dysfunction in one of these usually quickly progresses to dysfunction in all three.

To appraise brain function the physician must make a careful neurologic and mental status examination, but a few simple questions will elicit indications of the more urgent problems: Does the patient respond to me? Is he awake? Does he know where he is, how far he is from his home, what day it is, and about what time of the day it is? Is he responding appropriately to my presence, or is he struggling with and hostile to someone who is here to help him? If he is confused, hostile, or asleep and not easily roused to full alertness, then he may be a true emergency and the staff physician must be alerted.

Adequate evaluation of the respiratory system requires only a few simple observations. What is the patient's respiratory rate? A full minute should be counted. A rate under 12 or over 20 per minute should be considered a bright-red danger signal. All too often tachypnea is written off as "hyperventilation," and the correct diagnosis of pneumonia, metabolic acidosis, or subarachnoid hemorrhage is delayed. While the respiratory rate is counted, the regularity of respiration should be noted. A chaotic or cyclic respiratory pattern is cause for alarm. Volume of ventilation may be difficult to ascertain by watching the patient's chest or listening to it. It is easier to estimate the volume of air moved by placing a hand loosely over the patient's nose and mouth during respiration. Again, either a low or a high volume of ventilation is a serious sign of imminent disaster. The patient's color should be gauged, and if he is dusky gray or blue, especially about the tongue and lips, he is in danger. Finally, the patient may complain of being short of breath, choking, unable to get his breath, or unable to stop coughing long enough to breathe.

Problems involving the cardiovascular system may be signaled by the most awesome physical signs, such as no palpable pulse, or may present with a normal, healthy-appearing patient who says that his chest discomfort has now vanished. Chest pain or discomfort is ominous because of its association with sudden death and myocardial infarction.

The pulse and blood pressure, especially if taken both supine and seated or upright, provide a wealth of information. An irregular pulse, or one with a rate under 50 or over 120 is a danger sign par excellence. A low blood pressure (systolic BP of 100 plus patient's age will give a first approximation of the patient's blood pressure) or one that falls significantly when the patient stands is, of course, very dangerous. The mean blood pressure can be approximated by the diastolic BP plus one-third of the pulse pressure. This mean should not fall 10 mm Hg on standing. A fall of 10 mm is probably dangerous and one of 15 surely significant. This maneuver will pick up hypovolemia, one of the most common pathologic processes seen in an emergency room as a true emergency.

There is no such thing as a "little bit of shock." Shock is a serious problem. A drop in blood pressure due to bleeding indicates a loss of at least one-third of the total blood volume. Narcotics, of course, can add to the hypotension by vasodilation and should be avoided in a case such as this.

Fluid repletion must be done quickly with crystalloid or colloid or blood. Large intravenous channels are needed, and since the resistance of the tube is proportionate to its length, there is no place in resuscitation of a trauma victim for long-line catheters. A central venous pressure catheter is helpful, but it should be a short tube in the internal jugular or subclavian vein, if fluid is to be infused rapidly through this route. The resistance of a tube is also proportionate to the fourth power of its radius, so a large catheter with a diameter about twice that of a medium one can infuse fluids sixteen times as fast.

23

A 24-YEAR-OLD MAN was brought to the ER by ambulance. He
had placed a firecracker in his anus and lit it. The explosion brought
him to the attention of bystanders, and he was brought in with a
small amount of blood leaking from his anus. He had a past history
of many psychiatric hospitalizations for schizophrenia and for
"sexual deviancy." He had come to the emergency room previously
with self-inflicted razor cuts of the scrotum. He had been in the
state psychiatric hospital for two years for "child molestation."

On physical examination the patient appeared well. There was
a small mucosal tear of the anal canal and no further pathology on
proctoscopic examination. Vital signs were normal. He was referred
to the psychiatric unit for evaluation.

How does one treat rectal injuries?

What part of the treatment is most often overlooked?

We have removed from rectal ampullae a variety of foreign bodies, including pop bottles, razor blades, and electric vibrators. The trauma done to the rectum is often underestimated. A tear may lead to retroperitoneal abscess, which has a high mortality. Whenever doubt exists, we do a colostomy and drainage procedure. In this case the damage was limited to the anal canal and was trivial. Sitz baths alone were adequate therapy.

There is considerable rectal fascination in nonschizophrenics, and one ought not to jump to the diagnosis of schizophrenia in all patients who introduce foreign objects into the rectum. However, we seem to find that most of our rectal inserters are, in fact, long-standing schizophrenics. Evaluation of such patients must include attention to both ends. Careful proctoscopy must be done. Removal of large foreign bodies may require insertion of a gloved hand with near-general anesthesia. Preoccupation with the rectal lesion can cause the physician to forget to consult a psychiatrist, and this may be the most serious omission possible.

This incident was triggered by the patient's failure to take his antipsychosis medications, which resulted in the reactivation of his psychosis. Returning him to his usual therapy was enough to achieve control of his psychotic behavior.

A 39-YEAR-OLD WOMAN came to the emergency room complaining of abdominal pain and vomiting for two days following a day of rather heavy drinking. She denied any significant past ills but admitted that she would get an "acid stomach" if she drank two or more beers. On physical exam she appeared entirely normal except for slight diffuse abdominal tenderness. Blood pressure was 116/84 supine and 106/80 seated. Her pulse was 120 supine or seated. One ounce of Mylanta antacid gave her relief from pain, and a finger-stick hematocrit was 53%. A complete blood count and a set of electrolytes were sent to the lab but were lost there. After two hours the patient said she felt well and was sent home on a regimen of antacid, propoxyphene (Darvon) for pain, and fluids, with instructions to return if she remained ill.

Four days later she returned in severe distress. Her blood pressure was 75 systolic. Her abdomen was tense and tympanitic. Temperature was 38.6°C. An x-ray showed free air under the diaphragm. She was hyponatremic, hypokalemic, and dehydrated. Central venous pressure was zero, and the patient was treated with high-flow intravenous fluids. After four hours she was explored. The findings included a perforated duodenal ulcer, peritonitis, and several areas of near-necrotic bowel. Despite heroic emergency measures, *Escheria coli* and clostridial sepsis developed, and the patient died one week after exploration.

Had the ulcer perforated at the time of the patient's first ER visit?

How does one make the diagnosis of an acute abdomen requiring surgical attention?

24 DISCUSSION

We cannot tell retrospectively whether the patient's ulcer had perforated on her first admission. The tachycardia suggests that she was sicker than she seemed.

An acute abdomen can present in obscure ways, and the diagnosis can easily be missed. A physician with considerable diagnostic acumen may have had little experience with acute abdominal pain. Surgeons are usually the most sensitive to the subtle signs of an acute abdomen. In general, the cases we have missed were those not seen by a surgeon. Usually, the older patient, the alcoholic, the debilitated, diabetic, or leukemic patient, and the steroid-treated patient will be the ones to mask an acute abdomen. An upright film of the abdomen and a CBC might help, but whenever there is doubt, consult a surgeon.

The classic features of an acute abdomen are distention, rigidity, vomiting, and pain, and while all four need not be present in any particular acute abdominal problem, usually at least two are. Distention is often written off as unimportant by patient and physician alike by calling it "gas." There is a popular folk belief that most of the ills of mankind can be ascribed to "too much gas." Indeed, gaseous distention is a sign of underlying disease, not a cause. Rigidity occurs in patients with serious acute abdominal states such as pancreatitis, appendicitis, cholecystitis, or a perforated viscus. It is affected by awareness and often lessens when the patient's attention is diverted. The onset of pain before other symptoms may be the most important hint to the presence of acute abdomen.

A 50-YEAR-OLD MAN was involved in an auto accident. Seemingly unprovoked, he drove his car down a hillside into a creek. The car rolled over, and the man bounced about but stayed in the car. A police car arrived, and the officers extricated the patient. After the ambulance arrived, the attendant was able to learn from the patient that he was a diabetic. The patient was then brought to the emergency room, and the ambulance attendant told a passing nurse that he had a diabetic who had rolled his car. The nurse glanced at the patient and, deeming him "in not too bad shape," went on about her work in another room. The ambulance attendant returned to his ready room to watch television.

The patient became more confused, and by the time he was seen by a physician fifteen minutes later was stuporous and could give no history. The physician arrived with a blank encounter form and an ambulance trip report that stated only "auto accident — possible injuries." The patient had no obvious signs of head injury and no focal neurologic signs but was clearly confused and stuporous. Fortunately, a youth who was in the room, waiting for his girlfriend on the next bed to be sutured, remarked that the man was a diabetic: "I heard the ambulance driver say so." A blood sugar was drawn, and 50 ml of 50% glucose solution was given intravenously. The patient became much more alert, and the blood sugar was later reported at 30 mg per 100 milliliters.

What sort of information should one try to elicit from the ambulance crew, firemen, policemen, or other on-the-scene observers?

If focal neurologic signs developed in the patient, would that rule out hypoglycemia?

Is it true that most city hospital emergency-room patients carry cards saying, "I am not a diabetic, I am drunk."?

Patient history information is of great value to the emergency-room physician. All too often the patient is confused or comatose or becomes so shortly after arrival at the emergency room. Often no one is present who can give information about the patient. Relatives may never arrive at the emergency room even though they tell the ambulance attendant they are coming in, or they may leave the emergency room before the physician can talk with them.

We like our ambulance attendants to try to determine the following information and include it in the trip report for each case:

A. Trauma Patient
1. What happened before the event? Was the patient acting strange? Did he pass out, become confused, fall, become dizzy? Did he complain of any symptoms? Was he on any drugs or other treatment? Alcohol?
2. Description of event: If a weapon was involved, what size and sort? If a fall, how far and in what position? If an auto accident, was he seat-belted? Where was he seated? Was he thrown out? Did he hit any secondary objects?
3. What did he then do? Was he unconscious? Was there retrograde amnesia? Could he move his extremities? Did he complain of pain or shortness of breath? What has been the course of consciousness since the event?
4. Other information: Whom can we contact for further information regarding the accident (an observer of the event)? Whom for background on the patient? Is he on any drugs? Is he allergic to any drugs? Is he being cared for by a physician for any chronic illness? Name of physician? Who can help us in subsequent care of patient?
5. How does patient now feel? What hurts (the major injury may not be the most apparent)? Trouble breathing? Confusion? Amnesia? Weakness? Dizziness?

B. Nontrauma Patient
1. Describe major symptoms. A history taken by a neophyte tends to accept as important information the patient's own

diagnosis or suggested therapy: This must be bypassed and his symptoms elicited.

2. *Why now?* What happened to lead patient to pick this moment to seek help? Sometimes this is obvious, but if not, the question must be answered.

3. Is the patient being treated for chronic illness? Name of physician? What drugs is he taking (include over-the-counter medicines)? Any allergies to drugs? Who can give us more information? Who will help us care for him?

4. What events occurred (and when) during ride into ER?

Hypoglycemia may present in many ways. Confusion, anger, fighting, ataxia, anxiety, stupor, or focal neurologic findings all may be present in one or another diabetic. Hypoglycemia is indeed a medical emergency and should be treated promptly. The nurse involved in this case did not realize the significance of an auto accident for a person with diabetes.

Hypoglycemia may mimic alcohol intoxication and in a busy city hospital emergency room is often confused with alcohol intoxication. To further confuse the issue, alcoholics with depleted hepatic glycogen stores may develop hypoglycemia even without insulin or other drug therapy. One may always draw a blood sugar and a blood alcohol, but if the diagnosis of hypoglycemia is being entertained, there is almost never any harm in giving a bolus of sugar (orally in a conscious patient or intravenously in a comatose one). We usually give 25 gm of glucose intravenously and may repeat it once or twice. We start an intravenous infusion of 5% dextrose in water and keep the patient in the emergency room for several hours. The hypoglycemic action (especially with certain oral hypoglycemic drugs) may long outlast the effect of the glucose given, and the patient may lapse back into coma. Careful observation, oral sugar once awake, and instructions regarding future therapy are necessary.

Differentiating between a metabolic encephalopathy (e.g., hypoglycemia, anoxia or postanoxia, uremia, hyponatremia) and a traumatic encephalopathy (e.g., postconcussion, subdural hematoma) and a toxic encephalopathy (e.g., alcohol, sedative, other drugs) can test the most agile neurologist. The patient history, as in this case, can save the day.

It is not true that our alcoholic patients have cards identifying them as "drunk." However, many diabetics do fail to carry proper identification.

26 *

A 35-YEAR-OLD MAN had been drinking heavily until two days before he came to the emergency department. When he arrived he complained that he had become shaky and felt sick. He appeared slightly pale, had tremors, and was perspiring but afebrile. The man was alert and gave no evidence of hallucinations. He appeared somewhat dry. He was treated with intravenous fluids and sedation. During the next three hours he began to feel much better and lost his tremor to a large extent. He was discharged, but as he got out of the bed to leave, he collapsed on the floor. He was then found to be hypotensive, and his hematocrit was only 13%. Subsequent evaluation showed significant upper gastrointestinal bleeding — probably from a duodenal ulcer or an acute gastritis. The patient was hospitalized for further therapy.

In evaluating a withdrawing alcoholic, what history and physical examination data should be collected to rule out the most common serious associated illnesses?

If you think you are dealing with an upper GI bleeder, what should you do in the ER?

*Adapted from Platt, F. W., More than DTs. *Emergency Medicine* 4:167, January 1972. Used by permission of the publisher.

We have found the following workup very helpful in identifying patients who are withdrawing from alcohol but are too ill for a simple detoxification (drying-out) ward to handle. The serious diseases picked up include acute head trauma, acute or chronic subdural hematomas, epidural hematomas, pneumonia, tuberculosis, and severe hypovolemia.

Evaluation of Alcohol Withdrawal Patients

A. History
   1. Chief complaint — main symptom. Duration of Sx's.*
      Alleviating and worsening factors. COMMENT: These
      patients often cannot clarify this more than "sick."
   2. Drinking how much?_____ of what? _____
      Last drink when?_____ How long this binge?_____
      How long sober before?_____
      When last on detox ward?_____
   3. Smokes _____ packs/day.
      Cough _____ oz. _____(color) sputum/day.
      Tuberculosis history?_____Chest pain?_____
      Short of breath?_____
   4. Head trauma recently?_____
      Seizures? _____ Hallucinations?_____
   5. Vomiting blood? (how much) _____
      Black, tarry stools? _____
   6. Taking medications?_____ Allergic to medicines? _____
      Any other serious illnesses? _____
   7. Other: _____
B. Physical Exam
   BP_____ P_____ right arm, recumbent
   BP_____ P_____ right arm, standing or sitting
                           (check which)
   Temp_____ Respiration _____Weight _____
   HEENT —   (jaundice, evidence of head trauma)
   Neck, Nodes —
   Chest —
   *Symptoms.

Cardiovascular — (cardiomegaly, edema, gallops, . . .)
Abdomen —   (tenderness, liver size, . . .)
Rectal — Stool to hematest
Neurologic —   (gait, nystagmus, mental status)
C. Lab
Chest x-ray_____ CBC _____
Urinalysis _____ Blood alcohol _____

Upper GI bleeding is a life-threatening problem. We try to determine whether the patient is significantly hypovolemic, and if so expand his blood volume with saline or lactated Ringer's solution. We pass a nasogastric tube and, if any evidence of bleeding is obtained, initiate gastric lavage with iced saline. We obtain blood for typing and crossmatch at least 4 units of whole blood and do a hematocrit.

Patients with evidence of voluminous blood loss by history or of hypovolemia by examination are admitted, usually to the medical service. Tarry stools or a low hematocrit usually lead to admission. An occasional patient will complain of vomiting blood and will have normal vital signs without a postural change, a normal hematocrit, and negative stool and gastric aspirate. Such a patient may be sent home.

Lower GI bleeding usually presents with red blood passed by rectum. Proctoscopy should be done in the ER to locate the bleeding site and evaluate the rectal mucosa. Hemorrhoidal bleeding is, of course, most common and is usually less significant than bleeding from the rectum or higher.

A 54-YEAR-OLD ZOO KEEPER was bitten by a leopard. Some sort of illness had killed one leopard in the zoo, and the others were being treated with parenteral tetracycline prophylactically. The zoo keeper was trying to hold the leopard down for its shot when it bit him on the hand. He was seen in the employees' health clinic, where he was given a shot of tetanus toxoid. The following day he came to the ER complaining of a painful, swollen hand. He was afebrile. There were no red streaks on his arm, and he had only one small, nontender lymph node in the right axilla. There were two small, closed puncture wounds evident. The patient was taken to the operating room where incision and drainage were done under regional anesthesia. Copious pus was drained and cultured.

What organism is most likely to be cultured?

Should the patient be started on rabies vaccine?

Are any other animal bites handled differently?

Is it true that the bite of the leopard is the most dangerous known to man?

Leopards are unusual in having frequent bouts of *Escherichia coli* septicemia. One might thus expect an *E. coli* septic abscess. Nonetheless, the organism cultured was *Pasteurella multocida*. This organism is present in large amounts in the saliva of the domestic cat and often in that of dogs. Cat bites are notorious for rapid accumulation of pus and rapid swelling. Fortunately, *P. multocida* is very sensitive to almost any antibiotic and responds well to a ten-day course of penicillin, erythromycin, or tetracycline. One may occasionally do without incision and drainage if the drug is begun before a true abscess forms. In this case, initiation of antibiotic therapy one day earlier might have eliminated the need for surgery. Penicillin is probably the best first choice.

Rabies vaccination is not appropriate in this case. The question of rabies prophylaxis usually comes up in connection with a dog bite. Even then, unless considerable tissue damage has been done, especially on the head or neck, no therapy need be done if the animal can be observed. A rabid dog is a sick dog and will either die shortly or be so ill as to warrant sacrificing and autopsy. The city dogcatcher can be notified through the police and will handle the matter. We treat dog bites with copious irrigation, scrubbing with soap, debridement if needed, tetanus toxoid, and antibiotics. We generally do not suture such wounds.

Skunk and bat bites should be assumed to carry rabies and should be treated. The minimum recommended dosage of rabies vaccine is fourteen daily doses given subcutaneously with boosters ten and twenty days after the series. Antirabies serum can be given if rabies is strongly suspected and if the wound is on the head or neck or is extensive. This is horse serum, and sensitivity testing must be done first.

Human bites are probably the most serious that we see. They should be debrided and treated as described for dog bites. They must be observed closely and hospitalization urged at any sign of infection or gas formation in the tissues. Prophylactic antibiotics are appropriate with human bites and probably should be begun with parenteral procaine penicillin G (2.4 or 4.8 million units) plus oral penicillin V (500 mg qid).

A 51-YEAR-OLD MAN was brought to the emergency room by ambulance. He was found lying on the street, and one observer said that he may have had a seizure. On arrival in the ER, he had a pulse of 120, blood pressure 150/80, respiration rate 18, and was somnolent. He responded to deep pain by withdrawing but did not respond to voice commands. His right pupil was slightly larger than the left. He had no asymmetry of reflexes or tone, and plantar responses were flexor. "Doll's eyes" (oculocephalic responses) were not evaluated. He was given 50 gm of glucose (100 ml of 50% glucose solution) by vein, and blood sugar, BUN, and electrolyte samples were drawn. There was no improvement, and shortly there-after the patient had a generalized seizure during which he seemed to be looking to the right. A skull film showed a probable fracture, and a carotid arteriogram was done but was normal. The following laboratory data were then returned: a BUN of 3 mg per 100 ml, blood sugar of 480 mg per 100 ml (unfortunately drawn after the bolus of sugar was given), and electrolytes showing a sodium con-centration of 98 mEq/L, chloride 62 mEq/L, potassium 3.4 mEq/L, and bicarbonate 16 mEq/L. Treatment with 3% saline solution and KCl led to arousal and then pulmonary congestion. The patient was then admitted to the hospital.

What is the significance of unequal pupils after a seizure?

How low must the serum sodium be before ascribing seizures or confusion to it?

What causes hyponatremia?

28 DISCUSSION

Seizures may lead to unequal neurologic signs in the postictal period. Todd's paralysis or anisocoria are not unusual. The postictal findings may help define the focus of the seizures in the brain. In this case the physicians were concerned about the possibility of impending cerebral herniation due to a subdural or epidural hematoma, and an arteriogram was needed to rule out the presence of an evacuatable mass lesion. Subdural hematomas, however, rarely present with seizures.

The evaluation of a seizure patient should include blood sugar and serum sodium analyses. Hypoglycemia or hyponatremia (sodium concentration under 120 mEq/L) may cause seizures. The cause of hyponatremia is not always clear but usually includes excessive sodium loss or excessive water intake and may include an excessive, inappropriate antidiuretic hormone secretion. This has been associated with acute and chronic diseases of lung and brain. Young people may develop hyponatremia after vigorous exercise with heavy sweating and repletion of volume with water but not salt. They usually present first with muscle and abdominal cramps but may progress to seizures.

Needless to say, a blood sugar obtained after giving glucose has little value. A few seconds spent obtaining a sample before therapy would have been worthwhile.

A 24-YEAR-OLD WOMAN came to the emergency room complaining of vaginal bleeding. She had begun her periods at age 13; they had quickly become regular at about a 26 to 28-day interval and generally lasted 5 to 7 days. She had been pregnant twice, resulting in full-term deliveries one and four years ago. She now was generally well, with no fever or chills, and was on no medications. Three months prior to this visit she had had an intrauterine device (IUD) inserted. Her menstrual periods had subsequently been appearing about every 20 to 25 days and lasting 8 days with copious flow. The present menstrual flow was tapering off at the eighth day. She had noticed cramping with her period the first time after insertion of the IUD but not since.

On examination, the patient was afebrile, and her abdomen was nontender. Pelvic exam showed normal external genitalia, no pathology of Bartholin's glands, Skene's glands, or urethra, and a normal vaginal mucosa. The cervix was pink with a trickle of blood from the os. The uterus was only slightly tender, anterior, and normal in size. The adnexae were neither enlarged nor excessively tender. Rectal examination revealed no pathology; stool was brown. The cervix was cultured for gonorrhea after careful removal of the obvious blood. This culture later was reported to be negative.

What should you do with this patient?

Should the IUD be removed?

If the vaginal vault was noted to have copious amounts of creamy discharge, what should be done?

29 DISCUSSION

Intrauterine devices frequently cause heavy irregular bleeding for several months after insertion. Usually removal is not necessary. As in many cases of bleeding, vital signs should be checked to rule out significant volume loss, and a hematocrit should be obtained. Uterine cramping is frequent for up to one month after insertion of an IUD but usually can be treated with mild analgesics or "antispasmodics" such as phenobarbital and belladonna, one tablet every four hours, without need for removal of the IUD. Ordinary vaginal infections may be treated without removal of the IUD. If a discharge is present, it should be examined microscopically by placing some in saline on a slide with a cover slip. Yeast (monilia) and trichomonas protozoa are usually obvious. Culture for gonorrhea should be done and probably is a wise screening maneuver whenever a pelvic exam is done.

Oral contraceptives are often associated with breakthrough bleeding in the first three months of initiation of therapy or on change of drug or dosage. In general, patients should be urged to wait about three months after starting or changing therapy to see if nuisance symptoms disappear. If removal of an IUD or discontinuation of pills is necessary, the patient should be referred to the family planning clinic for alternate methods of contraception. For some patients pregnancy may be even worse than the presenting symptoms.

This patient may benefit from a one-month course of an oral estrogenic contraceptive such as norethynodrel and mestranol (as in Enovid-E) or ethinyl estradiol (Demulen) with the IUD in place. This may terminate the bleeding problem.

A 26-YEAR-OLD MAN came to the emergency room complaining of a cold. He felt that a shot of penicillin would clear him up. He claimed a cough productive of about one shotglass (2 oz.) of green-yellow sputum daily for the past week. The cough was associated with a ripping substernal pain that he said felt like he was "coming apart with the cough." He smoked about one-and-one-half packs of cigarettes a day but commented that he seldom finished a cigarette and that his friends bummed many cigarettes from him, contributing to that total. In describing his smoking he said that he smoked "not too much." He also commented on a stuffy head but denied earache, ear drainage, or severe headaches. He noted mild hoarseness. He felt that shortness of breath was not a problem but that recently any activity was causing coughing spells that were hard to stop. Deep breathing also would provoke such a spell, and the coughing frequently led to retching. He denied drug allergies.

On physical exam, the patient had a temperature of 37.5°C orally, a respiratory rate of 18, a pulse of 94, and a blood pressure of 130/84 in the right arm when seated. His pharynx was a bit red, but his tympanic membranes were normal. He had no tenderness over the maxillary sinuses or under the supraorbital ridge. His voice was slightly rough, and he sniffled frequently. As he took a deep breath, a vibratory sensation was palpable bilaterally over the middle ribs laterally. With a stethoscope, coarse rhonchi were audible bilaterally. When asked to cough, he produced a few milliliters of yellow sputum.

What is a "cold"?

What does this patient have?

How would you treat this patient?

The popular term "cold" has no exact medical significance but usually is equated with a viral upper respiratory infection. "Upper respiratory" is usually taken to mean larynx and above, leaving the trachea, bronchi, bronchioles, and lungs to the "lower respiratory" system. Thus, upper respiratory symptoms include headache, earache, ear drainage, tinnitus, rhinorrhea, stuffy head, sore throat, pain on swallowing, swollen cervical nodes, and loss of voice. Lower respiratory symptoms are chiefly three: cough, shortness of breath, and chest pain. These are, of course, more significant than upper respiratory symptoms. Upper respiratory infections are either viral or bacterial. Viral upper respiratory infections (URIs) include mononucleosis. Bacterial URIs include streptococcal infections and, less commonly, hemophilus, meningococcus, and diphtheria infections. In general, penicillin is good therapy if a bacterial URI is diagnosed, since the organism is usually streptococcus. A throat culture should be done when the patient complains of a sore throat or earache or has sinus tenderness. Severe hoarseness to the point of aphonia associated with local laryngeal tenderness may be the presentation of acute epiglottitis in an adult. This is a rare bacterial URI and deserves hospitalization. Usually laryngitis is a viral infection.

This patient, of course, has a *lower* respiratory infection. A chest x-ray may reveal bronchopneumonia but will probably be normal. The diagnosis is bronchitis, and the etiology may be either viral or bacterial. With yellow or green sputum we usually treat bronchitis with an antibiotic and usually pick tetracycline or ampicillin.

More importantly, the patient should be told to stop smoking during this illness (and preferably thereafter). He should be encouraged to drink copious amounts of nonalcoholic fluids and to obtain some means of inhaling a high-humidity atmosphere to aid him in bringing up sputum. The easiest means is usually to spend thirty to sixty minutes twice a day in his bathroom with the hot water in the tub or shower on, filling the room with steam. The patient should not be *in* the hot water (to avoid a burn) but should remain in the room with windows and doors closed. Many patients will request cough medicines, but the patient with a productive cough or a fever should not be given cough suppressants such as codeine: He needs his cough to drain the purulent secretions. If given at all, cough suppressants should be limited to nighttime use to allow sleep. Sputum gram stains or cultures have been of little help to us in acute bronchitis.

31

A 50-YEAR-OLD MAN was brought to the emergency room by ambulance. He had been found lying in the street unconscious. There was no obvious evidence of trauma.

On arrival the man was comatose. He appeared unkempt, unshaven, and dirty. There was a distinct alcohol odor mingled with several less well-defined odors. He moved away from painful stimuli but would not respond to verbal communications. Vital signs included a pulse rate of 100, respiratory rate of 15, blood pressure of 160/90, and temperature of 37.5°C rectally. He had positive oculocephalic reflexes, commonly termed "doll's eyes" movements (on tilting his head to the right, his eyes briefly moved to the left, and vice versa). His muscle tone was normal throughout. Deep tendon reflexes were symmetric, although ankle jerks could not be elicited. The plantar responses were flexor. Respiration was regular. There was no evidence of head trauma, and pupils were equal. An intravenous route was established, and 50 ml of 50% glucose solution was given. No response was noted. The patient was felt to be in alcoholic stupor. Blood sugar, set of electrolytes, and blood alcohol analyses were ordered. The patient was laid supine on the bed and tied down to prevent him from falling. He was spreadeagled, tied with gauze restraints, and left to sober up. Two hours later he was less asleep; he vomited and aspirated some of the vomitus. He did not suffer a respiratory arrest but was thought to have an aspiration pneumonitis and was admitted to the medical ward.

What is the preferred position in which to place comatose patients?

How do you treat aspiration?

Coma position should insure patency of the airway. If the patient vomits (not uncommon in an unconscious patient), the emesis should pour out by gravity and not remain in the pharynx to cause obstruction or be aspirated into the lungs. The standard position is semiprone, semilateral decubitus with the top arm pulled down, the head forward, and the mouth down and preferably off the edge of the bed. Vomitus will then tend to pour off the bed. The patient can be tied in such a position and be relatively safe.

Of course, nothing is better than close observation, but all too often a patient is well observed in an ER until a patient in worse shape arrives, and then attention is diverted from the first patient. Some emergency units have attached observation wards with monitoring facilities and a separate nursing staff. Unless such an intensive care observation unit is maintained, observation in the ER system may be inadequate. Since many seriously ill patients recover well within twelve hours, and since most city hospitals are continually short of beds, the use of such a unit seems essential.

Observation should include signs of increasing intracranial pressure (checking pupils for size and reactivity, arousability, pulse, and blood pressure). A comatose patient who is not clearly more alert in four hours should be admitted to the hospital.

Once a patient has aspirated, severe chemical pneumonitis will develop unless therapy is immediate and correct: Gastric acid is an irritant that produces inflammation. A large dose of intravenous steroids, such as 500 to 1000 mg of hydrocortisone or 20 to 40 mg of dexamethasone, should be given as soon as aspiration is suspected. Minutes are important, and no time should be lost. If solid particulate material was aspirated, bronchoscopy should be done as soon as possible. Antibiotics are usually begun, although their use is perhaps less clear than the steroids.

32

A 23-YEAR-OLD MAN came to the emergency room complaining of shortness of breath, fatigue, and coughing up blood. He claimed he had had these symptoms for about ten months and denied any remarkable recent worsening. He admitted smoking one pack of cigarettes daily. His cough produced about one ounce of almost pure blood daily. He could do very little without dyspnea and had quit his job about one year earlier because of fatigue and dyspnea. He slept flat but several times a week awoke with choking and walked about the house, drank water, even went outdoors before settling back in bed. He denied any chest pain and had no history of rheumatic fever or heart murmur.

This night he called for help when he awoke from an afternoon nap in a state of panic. He was confused and terrified. The confusion quickly disappeared, but the panic remained. He had recently been having marital difficulties and was separated from his wife. In the past there had been several episodes of panic but none as severe as today's.

On physical examination, the patient appeared anxious and tremulous. His pulse was 100, respiration 24, blood pressure 150/80, and temperature 37.5°C. His chest was clear, jugular venous pressure normal, and he had no edema. Pulses were normal. His cardiac impulse was forceful but not sustained and was localized at the fourth intercostal space in the midclavicular line. He had no abnormal gallops, a loud S_1 and S_2, and a faint short systolic murmur at the aortic area. On being asked to cough, he produced bloody saliva by sucking at a bleeding gum about a carious tooth. He had no adenopathy and no thyromegaly. The patient appeared otherwise normal. A chest x-ray was normal.

What should next be done for this patient?

In what order should organic and psychiatric symptoms be pursued in the ER?

This young man presented clear organic-sounding symptoms and clear emotional symptoms. Of the two, the reason for his arrival at the emergency room was the acute panic, and this should be attacked. Physicians are often loath to approach psychiatric problems due to their own insecurities. Nonetheless, the ER must attend primarily to the problems bringing the patient in *today* as opposed to last week or next week. Often, as in this case, a combined approach works best. This man was assured that he had several problems, that his lungs and heart seemed to have nothing *serious* wrong with them but that he should be seen again in the medical clinic. He was told that an interview with one of the psychiatry staff was essential and that his teeth needed attention. He was given some mild sedation (Valium, 5 mg 2 to 4 times a day), and after an initial psychiatric interview was calmer and returned home.

This case was grossly unfinished as the patient left the ER. However, several things were begun. An appraisal had been made of possible life-threatening cardiac or pulmonary disease and none found. The importance of the emotional features of the illness had been stressed to the patient and arrangements made for followup. The obvious features of malingering (sucking on a bleeding mouth lesion and claiming the bloody saliva as hemoptysis) did not go unnoticed, but the patient properly was not punished for this. In fact, this unusual behavior should be viewed as a cry for help — producing more symptoms in order to be heard.

In general, one should work up what appears to be most prominent. A barber once told me that his technique was "to cut off whatever sticks out." This is the most fruitful ER approach — that is, examine whatever sticks out. If psychopathology stares you in the face, evaluate it first, not after a major organic workup proves negative. Usually a combined approach is needed. Fear of labeling the patient a neurotic should not lead the doctor to avoid dealing with emotional symptoms that the patient desperately wants to discuss.

33

A 20-YEAR-OLD WOMAN was brought to the emergency room on a Saturday night with a laceration of the wrist. She had cut her wrist with a razor blade and was brought to the ER by ambulance. The ambulance attendant had placed a pressure dressing on the superficial wrist laceration, which was bleeding slowly. The patient was relatively uncommunicative but admitted she felt depressed.

During the preceding eighteen months the woman had spent over thirteen months hospitalized on several psychiatric wards with the diagnosis of depression. During the preceding week she had appeared at the Denver General Hospital emergency room five times. She had been discharged from the psychiatry inpatient unit on Tuesday and that evening returned to the ER with slashed wrists. The wounds were irrigated and sutured, and she was referred to the psychiatry team, who interviewed her and judged her to be not suicidal. Two days later, on Thursday, she arrived at the ER to discuss her worsening depression with the psychiatry team. After her interview she went out, only to return four hours later with a new laceration of the left wrist. On Friday she was brought in with a presumed overdose of aspirin, Librium, and Thorazine. She refused to wait for a physician to see her and left within an hour of her arrival. The emergency room had been very busy with major trauma cases, and both nurses and physicians viewed her as a nuisance rather than as a challenging new problem. On Saturday night she returned with her latest laceration. She was again sutured and referred to the psychiatry team. She announced that she was now under the care of an outside private psychiatrist. When he was called, he responded by stating that she was no suicide risk and that he was getting disgusted with her. Her parents had both killed themselves when she was 3 years old.

Is this patient suicidal?

What is she getting from the emergency room?

One of the ER physicians claims that the patient is in the running for the "Turkey of the Year Award." How do you believe she should be handled?

A successful suicide is by definition a disastrous event. In general, when a patient admits to depression, he should be queried about suicidal thoughts or plans. These should be taken seriously and a vigorous effort made to help the patient.

Viewing the gamut of patients who have made a suicide attempt and failed, one finds some with serious depression and desire to kill themselves and others with far less emotional distress who intended a mere gesture or an appeal for help, love, attention, or even punishment. Unfortunately serious intent does not always ensure success, and a mere gesture may accidentally be fatal. In general, psychiatrists tend to put the most effort into aiding suicidally de-pressed patients and not into working with people they judge to be immature gesturers. This patient is probably going to die by her own hand eventually, but any one attempt is not likely to be a serious one.

This patient exemplifies an extremely difficult ER problem. It is not clear what she is getting from the ER, but it is hard to believe that she is in any way getting assistance. She has been labeled a "chronic underdoser." Harassing the ER staff seems to be part of a destructive game she plays, destructive to her and to those super-ficially appearing to help her. At the very least, she is crying wolf too often and probably will not be heard when she cries the last time. She is becoming the victim of considerable ER staff hostility — perhaps indeed what she is trying to provoke. She interrupts and dilutes the care of other patients and makes the staff aware of its abject failure in dealing with her.

No one has been able to find a satisfactory approach to this sort of patient. Eventually she will probably be committed to the state psychiatric hospital. If indeed she is depressed, it is not the classic depression of a compulsive person. It appears to be more a depression of a lost soul with no hope, no successes, and no clear purchase on life. She does nothing well, not even suicide attempts. She has a meaningless life, and her more or less pathological involvement with the ER may be all the human contact she can tolerate or obtain. An apocryphal tale says that for a similar patient a collection was taken up one night by the ER staff. The collection bought a one-way bus ticket to a city 600 miles away and temporarily stopped the patient's visits to the ER.

A 72-YEAR-OLD MAN was brought to the emergency room because he had become faint at a bowling alley. On arrival at the ER he felt well. He was placed in the cardiac resuscitation room because that night it possessed the only working electrocardiograph. On examination he denied faintness, shortness of breath, or chest pain. He was being cared for by an outside physician and was on no medications. He believed that he had had a "heart attack" five years earlier that consisted of "auricular fibrillation."

His blood pressure was 110/70. His pulse was counted at 104 and was noted to be irregular, an apical pulse of 120 was noted. He had no edema, rales, or jugular venous pressure increase. He had carotid bruits but no heart murmurs. There was no evidence of cardiomegaly. The diagnostic ECG was normal except for the presence of atrial fibrillation.

While the patient was resting, still attached to the ECG monitor, he noted an unusual formation on the monitor oscilloscope and called it to the attention of the physician and ambulance attendant in the room. The formation appeared to be five ventricular beats in a row. These ended spontaneously and did not reappear. A defibrillator paddle was coated with electrode paste and placed under the patient's upper back. The other paddle was coated, and the capacitor charged with 400 watt seconds. An intravenous injection of lidocaine, 100 mg, was given. The patient's physician was contacted. He agreed to take over the patient's care if he could be transferred to a nearby private hospital but questioned the wisdom of moving him at that time.

Did this patient have a run of ventricular tachycardia?

How do you treat ventricular tachycardia?

What might have led to this patient's arrhythmias?

Ventricular tachycardia (VT) is usually a life-threatening arrhythmia because of the likelihood of its proceeding to ventricular fibrillation. In the ER it should always be assumed to be a disastrous arrhythmia and not the "benign ventricular tachycardia" that is often noted in coronary care units. Treatment should be rapid. It should begin with a brisk blow to the midsternal area. If that is unsuccessful, it should be followed by a synchronized direct current shock. This may be given at a low level, such as 20 watt seconds. If ineffective, higher levels of shock should be used. If an intravenous line is in place, 100 mg of lidocaine may be tried before or after the first shock.

In this case the patient converted spontaneously after a brief run of five ventricular beats. One could question whether five beats make a ventricular tachycardia, but a more important question is whether this was indeed VT or just aberration of conduction through the ventricles from a supraventricular tachycardia. There can be clues to aberration. Without visible P waves and with a basically irregular supraventricular rhythm (atrial fibrillation) one must look for:

1. A variable coupling interval to preceding beat — favoring aberration rather than ventricular beats.
2. A right bundle branch block pattern — favoring aberration slightly.
3. A deformed beat terminating a short R-to-R cycle preceded by a long cycle — suggesting aberration (but also often present with ectopic beats).
4. Runs of bigeminy — suggesting ectopy.

In this case the absence of a written record to study with these criteria in mind makes things more difficult. However, it is not wise to observe a patient too long to secure evidence which may be diagnostic for the physician but lethal for the patient. Lidocaine should be given here intravenously in a 100-mg bolus and followed by a lidocaine drip at 2 to 4 mg per minute.

Patients with myocardial infarctions may or may not have serious arrhythmias. On the other hand, a patient with life-threatening arrhythmias may not have had an infarction even though he has atherosclerotic coronary artery disease. Coronary artery disease may present with sudden death, myocardial infarction, self-limiting or benign arrhythmias, congestive heart failure, or angina pectoris. These may occur in combination or singly. With no clear history of pain nor an ECG diagnostic of infarction, we cannot yet say whether this patient had a myocardial infarction. However, he surely should be hospitalized. His atrial fibrillation is probably a recent change and may be responsible for his faintness. He may have had a brief but more serious arrhythmia at the bowling alley. His blood pressure is probably low and may be related to the arrhythmia or to the cause of the arrhythmia. Pulmonary embolism shoud be searched for as a cause of the atrial fibrillation. Transportation to another hospital should not be done at this time due to the inherent instability of the patient's situation. If this patient has been on digitalis, digitoxicity should be considered as another possible cause of his various arrhythmias.

The fact that this patient diagnosed his own ventricular tachycardia should not lessen its serious import for us. However, we should be doing the monitoring and should not have to rely on the patient to do this. At no time should his monitoring be unattended, from arrival in the ER to the coronary care unit.

A 44-YEAR-OLD MAN came to the emergency room complaining of chest pain after a fall down stairs four hours earlier while going to work. He had begun to hurt then, and the pain was worst at the right lower rib cage. He also hurt over the right buttock, where he had bounced down several steps. He noted pain in the chest on breathing deeply. He had smoked about one pack of cigarettes daily for about thirty years and always had a morning cough. Alcohol intake was not commented on.

On physical examination, the patient had marked tenderness over the right fifth through tenth ribs, maximal in the midaxillary line. His chest was clear to auscultation. He was afebrile, and otherwise normal.

X-ray pictures were taken, and no hip fracture or pulmonary infiltrates were seen. The patient had several lateral rib fractures. After his chest was painted with benzoin, 3-inch adhesive tape was applied from past the anterior midline around the painful hemithorax to a point past the vertebrae posteriorly. The tape was applied in overlapping strips to cover the hemithorax from the fourth to the eleventh ribs. The patient was given 20 tablets of APC with ½ grain of codeine and told to take one every four hours as needed for pain. He felt much better after the taping and thanked the physician.

Two days later the patient returned with more pain and a fever. Examination showed decreased breath sounds, rales, and wheezes at the right lung base. His temperature was 38.0°C orally, and he was otherwise normal. A chest x-ray showed an extensive right lower lobe pneumonia. He was admitted to the hospital for therapy.

Was the pneumonia an obligatory complication of the rib fractures?

What should have been done differently?

35 DISCUSSION

An effective cough, an effective muco-ciliary apparatus, and adequate local ventilation are all parts of maintaining the health of the lung. When these three mechanisms or other resistance phenomena are subverted, pneumonia is more likely. Smokers have considerable suppression of the ciliary activity in their bronchi and may not clear bacteria and debris from the lungs in the usual fashion. A cough may be essential. Codeine suppresses cough easily and may have been instrumental in the pneumonia development. The splinting induced by pain may be considerable, but taping adds to this and decreases local ventilation. This patient should have been urged to stop smoking, codeine probably should not have been used, and a nerve block extending above and below the involved ribs should have been done rather than taping.

The pneumonia rate is high in smokers who have fractured ribs, and the pain problem is difficult to deal with. This patient's alcohol intake was not discussed with him. Alcohol suppresses host defenses in several ways, including suppression of the bone marrow resulting in a leukopenia and suppression of the pulmonary muco-ciliary apparatus. If he was indeed a drinker, he should have been urged to abstain after his rib fractures. Finally, the actual fall down stairs was not defined clearly enough. Why and how did he fall down stairs? Had he been faint? Dizzy? Drunk? The event before the event bringing him to the ER (the fall) may be the most important part of his illness.

"Prophylactic" antibiotic therapy should be used in this sort of case to treat the bronchitis and avoid development of pneumonia.

A 30-YEAR-OLD MAN was brought to the emergency room by ambulance. He was described by the ambulance attendant as confused and probably drunk. He was noted to be absent without leave from a local private psychiatric hospital where he had been on therapy for alcoholism and had been on disulfiram (Antabuse) for one week. Today he had left the hospital and had drunk one quart of wine. Feeling ill, he went to a nearby police car and asked for assistance.

On arrival at the emergency room, the patient was observed to be uncooperative, lobster red in color, and to have a tachycardia of 140 beats per minute and a systolic blood pressure of 70 mm Hg. His chest was clear; his heart seemed normal except for the tachycardia; and he seemed otherwise normal. Rectal exam revealed brown stool that was negative when tested for occult blood. There was no obvious evidence of trauma. His jugular venous pressure seemed normal or low. His skin was warm and dry.

He was given 2000 ml of normal saline solution intravenously over sixty minutes. A chest x-ray and an ECG were done; they were normal. One gram of ascorbic acid (vitamin C) was given intravenously, and the patient lost his flush. The blood pressure moved up to 110 systolic by the end of his first liter of intravenous fluids. He left the ER four hours later feeling much better.

What causes hypotension in the alcohol-Antabuse reaction?

How should it be treated?

What does the vitamin C do?

Hypotension is a cardinal sign of a serious disease state and should be attacked vigorously. To do so one needs certain parameters of blood volume and extracellular fluid volume. Some of these were not obtained in this case. Most important are blood pressure and pulse in supine and erect positions, an estimate of the central venous pressure, weight, hematocrit, BUN, and serum sodium levels. With these one can attempt to distinguish among the three main mechanisms of hypotension. Cardiogenic shock usually is accompanied by an elevation of the venous pressure. Of course hypotension from any cause may lead to insufficient coronary artery perfusion and secondary pump failure. Hypovolemia due to bleeding into fracture sites, the GI tract, the peritoneum, retroperitoneum or externally will lead to hypotension when about 30% of the blood volume is lost. Water and salt may be lost externally or simply moved out of the vascular compartment, as is thought to be the case in alcohol-Antabuse reactions. Finally, vascular collapse due to adrenal insufficiency, sepsis, hypoxia, or drugs can lead to hypotension. Treatment of vascular collapse or hypovolemia is similar — rapid infusions of large amounts of crystalloids, colloid, or blood. A solution of 5% dextrose in water is a poor fluid for this purpose, and we usually start with normal saline solution or lactated Ringer's solution.

Antabuse interferes in some way with the metabolism of alcohol. It causes a pile-up of acetaldehyde, an oxidation product of alcohol, presumably by blocking the enzyme acetaldehyde dehydrogenase. Acetaldehyde can mimic some of the features of the alcohol-Antabuse reaction but *not* the hypotension, so it is not in itself enough to explain the reaction.

The reasons for use of vitamin C are obscure, but it seems to lessen the symptoms of the alcohol-Antabuse reaction. Some alcoholics even take oral vitamin C to "counteract the Antabuse" before drinking.

A 34-YEAR-OLD MAN was brought to the emergency room by ambulance. He had gone home after work and told his wife he would try to take a nap. She heard some noises in the bedroom and found him in the midst of a seizure. He bit his cheeks, jerked his arms and legs, and frothed at the mouth. She called an ambulance, which brought him to the ER. During the ride to the hospital he had a second generalized seizure. He had been generally well in the past but had a history of four seizures on one day five years ago. A diagnostic workup then had included brain scan, skull films, and an EEG; all were normal. At that time seizure medication was begun with Dilantin and phenobarbital. He took his medication for less than a year, then discontinued the drugs with no apparent ill effects. He smoked one pack of cigarettes daily and drank 2 to 4 ounces of whiskey most days. He was a public relations officer for one of the nearby police forces and had been working regularly with no signs of illness. He had suffered no recent head trauma and was on no other drugs.

The patient was stuporous on arrival at the ER. He seemed to struggle somewhat against those working with him. He had no focal abnormalities of tone or reflexes but, of course, strength and sensation could not be evaluated well. His blood pressure was 160/100 and pulse 100. He was afebrile. While he was being examined, he had two more brief seizures. Each began with generalized tonic-clonic movements and chewing, frothing mouthings. He did not waken between seizures.

The patient was given 10 mg of Valium intravenously and then 100 mg of phenobarbital intramuscularly. His seizures stopped. About ten minutes after the fourth seizure he was noted to have a respiratory rate of about 35. An arterial blood-gas sample was obtained, and the results were called to the ER thirty minutes later.

The pO_2 was 100 mm Hg (Denver has a barometric pressure of 630 mm Hg with a normal arterial pO_2 of 75 ± 10 mm Hg). The pCo_2 was 14 mm Hg and the pH 6.80 with a base excess of negative 16 mEq/L. A repeat pH was obtained at that time as well as serum acetone, serum salicylate, BUN, and a urinalysis. The repeat pH was 7.20, and all other studies were normal. Within two hours the patient was awake, but he could add no new information to the history. He was returned to phenobarbital and diphenylhydantoin and given an appointment in the neurology clinic.

What was wrong with this patient?

How low can the pH get following seizures?

What causes of a severe metabolic acidosis should be considered in this case?

This patient was in status epilepticus. This is defined as continuous seizure activity over five minutes or several seizures without regaining consciousness between them. This must be treated, and therapy usually consists of intravenous Valium or barbiturate or Dilantin or a combination thereof. Status epilepticus is life-threatening and must be stopped. Focal seizures or those with intermittent awake periods are not so serious, and one need not rush to treat them parenterally. Diazepam and amobarbital will stop a seizure but not prevent further ones, so the patient must also be given other anticonvulsant therapy.

When arterial pH samples are drawn soon after a seizure, we find it not uncommon for levels to be as low as 7.2. This patient's pH was extremely low at 6.8 and probably was due to considerable lactic acidosis following several hypoxic periods with his several fits. About 30% of our patients who have arterial pH's determined within thirty minutes of a seizure have a pH below 7.2; 15% are below 7.0.

Other causes of metabolic acidosis, such as ketoacidosis (usually diabetic but occasionally in a nondiabetic withdrawing alcoholic), or renal or exogenous drugs, must be considered.

In this case the clinical setting suggests the diagnosis of lactic acidosis, and the other etiologies can be ruled in or out by obtaining serum ketone, BUN, urine pH, serum salicylate, and blood alcohol analyses.

38

A 63-YEAR-OLD WOMAN was being driven to see her ophthal-
mologist when her car was hit from the right side by another auto-
mobile. The patient was not seat-belted and did not have high
seat backs in her car. While ricocheting about in the car, she hit
her head on the dashboard and was thrown into her brother and
back. After the car stopped, she got out, stood up, cried out, and
collapsed. An ambulance was called, and on arrival the attendants
felt no pulse and noted no respiration.

The patient was brought to the emergency room, with an attempt
at cardiac massage and respiration by face mask and bag in progress.
On arrival at the ER, her trachea was intubated by the oral route,
and self-inflating bag respiration was continued. Her pulse became
palpable, and a blood pressure of 70/40 was noted. Her central
venous pressure was measured by an internal jugular vein catheter
and was noted to be under 6 centimeters. Her pulse was 120 per
minute. Both pupils were large on arrival and became small shortly
thereafter. She seemed to have no asymmetries of tone or reflexes,
and no pathologic reflexes were present. She had a large laceration
across the forehead. Her chest and abdomen seemed normal. Two
large intravenous routes were established, and a Foley catheter was
placed in the bladder. A nasogastric tube was placed. A chest film,
skull films, abdominal films, and views of pelvis and femurs were
normal. An electrocardiogram was normal.

An abdominal tap was done and the abdomen irrigated with saline
solution. It returned clear fluid. The patient remained unconscious,
and a right carotid arteriogram was done. It appeared normal.
Blood pressure dropped to 50 systolic. Isoproterenol was begun,
and fluids were infused more rapidly. The blood pressure did not
change, and she was switched to Levarterenol. With this therapy
her blood pressure increased to 90 systolic. Her arterial pH was

7.35, and her arterial pO_2 was 85 mm Hg. She was admitted to the surgical intensive care unit, and her scalp laceration was sutured. During the next five days she had several cardiac arrests from which she was resuscitated. She died on the fifth day of hospitalization.

When do you do a carotid arteriogram in an unconscious patient?

Why was the patient hypotensive?

Is hypotension usually a feature of severe head trauma?

Once a traumatized unconscious patient develops any lateralizing signs, he deserves an arteriogram to search for a localized collection of blood that could be evacuated. In this case the persistent unconsciousness argued for such study even in the absence of lateralizing signs. There may be epidural, subdural, or intracerebral hematomas that need evacuation. As intracerebral pressure increases due to enlargement of a mass such as a hematoma, many neurologic changes may ensue, of which the most important is progressive loss of consciousness. As the alert patient becomes lethargic, then stuporous (rousable by voice even if his responses are inappropriate) then semicomatose and comatose, he should be considered a possible candidate for emergency neurosurgery. An endotracheal tube must be in place and ventilation assured. Some method should be tried to avoid brain edema. We usually give 100 to 300 gm (about 2 to 3 gm per kg of body weight) of Mannitol intravenously, occasionally give 10 mg of dexamethasone intravenously with 4 mg every six hours subsequently. We hyperventilate the unconscious patient. An indwelling urethral catheter is necessary to cope with the Mannitol-induced diuresis. Heart failure or renal failure contraindicates use of Mannitol.

The most remarkable feature in this case was the hypotension. Hypotension is almost never due to head injury. Characteristically, the patient with a head injury has a bradycardia and systolic hypertension with a wide pulse pressure. Hypotension should lead to a search for blood loss in the chest, abdomen, GI tract, retroperitoneum, or externally. In rare instances an infant can accumulate enough blood in a subdural hematoma to render him hypovolemic and hypotensive. An adult who has head injuries and hypotension needs a vigorous search for myocardial infarction, hypoxia, or occult blood loss. A search was made with this patient, but no such explanation was found. After death, an autopsy revealed multiple hemorrhages of the medulla and cerebrum. The lateral whipsawing blow probably severely traumatized her brain stem and led to damage at the medulla. Blood pressure regulation, of course, depends on a functioning brain stem.

A 54-YEAR-OLD WOMAN came to the emergency room complaining of pain on urinating over a period of several hours. She was urinating almost every thirty minutes and noted the urine to be red. She had had many past episodes of similar suprapubic and low back pain with passage of urine. A total abdominal hysterectomy had been done ten years earlier for "pelvic relaxation." Cystoscopy had been done five years earlier with a diagnosis of trigonitis but no evidence of obstruction. Several intravenous pyelograms (IVP's) had been done in the past and were normal.

On physical examination the patient was observed to be obese; she had a blood pressure of 174/110 and a temperature of 37.5°C orally. There was no costovertebral angle tenderness, and her abdomen was normal. No rectal or pelvic examination was done.

A urinalysis showed protein 2+, over 50 RBC's and over 50 WBC's per high-power field of spun sediment. A urine culture was done and later showed over 100,000 colonies of *Escherichia coli* per milliliter. All antibiotics tested were effective against the organism in vitro. The diagnosis then considered was hemorrhagic cystitis. She was placed on ampicillin, 500 mg orally qid for ten days, and pyridium, 100 mg tid for three days. Another IVP was scheduled and done the next day. It was normal. The patient was referred to the urology clinic. Despite her referral, she returned to the ER ten days after her first visit, now complaining of back pain and chills. She admitted to not taking her ampicillin regularly. She was afebrile but did now have left flank tenderness. Her repeat urinalysis showed about 4 RBC's and WBC's per high-power field; there was no more proteinuria. She was given more ampicillin and urged to take it as directed.

What is the most common reason for failure of drug therapy?

How should followup care be arranged for patients with urinary tract infections?

When should an IVP be done in patients with urinary tract symptoms?

What is a significant white blood cell count in a urinalysis?

It should not be surprising that the primary reason drug therapy fails is the patient's failure to take the drug. Most patients will do poorly at following directions when given only one drug, and the failure rate goes up as the number of prescriptions given increases. In general, one should try to limit therapy to a single drug. If several drugs or procedures are being advised, one should clearly define expectations and plans for the patient. It must be clear that he understands the plan, and that is best ascertained by asking him to recite it back to you.

Most patients who present with urinary tract symptoms at the ER have disease limited to the urethra or bladder. A surprising number (perhaps 20%) have some pyuria but no bacilluria and recover with or without antibiotics in the same three to seven days. Of the remainder, most have cystitis and respond well to a ten-day course of Sulfa or tetracycline or ampicillin. If a urinary tract infection (UTI) is diagnosed, the patient should be brought back in two to three days to check on the culture results, in vitro sensitivities, and clinical improvement. If the antibiotic is appropriate, the pyuria or hematuria should be nearly cleared in two days. A repeat urinalysis at this stage will clearly indicate a need to do more bacteriologic searching or to continue on the same regimen. Dysuria should clear in twenty-four hours.

Any evidence of renal involvement in a UTI (such as flank pain, high fever, or costovertebral-angle tenderness) should suggest an IVP. In addition, an IVP with postvoiding films should be done as part of a urologic workup in cases of repeated urinary tract infection. We usually work up a male with his second infection and a female with her third. Cystoscopy is appropriate at this stage, and so a referral to the urology clinic is needed. If gross hematuria is present, referral for cystoscopy is best even with a "first infection."

It is not clear how much leukocytosis in the urine constitutes pyuria. Women may have up to 5 WBC per high-power field with no infection, but in men even a few WBC may be significant.

Therapy with appropriate antibiotics should probably extend ten to fourteen days for cystitis and about twenty days for pyelonephritis.

Recurrent urethritis or cystitis in postmenopausal women may be associated with atrophic vaginal mucosa due to estrogen lack. Treatment with estrogens (e.g., Premarin, 2.5 mg daily for fifteen days, then cyclically 1.25 mg daily for twenty-five days of each month) improves the status of vaginal and urethral mucosa and decreases the incidence of infections.

40

A 48-YEAR-OLD MAN was brought to the emergency room by police car. His wife had called the police because he seemed confused and disoriented. He had been sitting in the bathroom brandishing a butcher knife and worrying about someone "coming for him." A mental health hold was placed, and he was brought to the ER.

On initial evaluation the following vital signs were obtained: blood pressure 130/90, pulse 120, temperature 37.6°C. He was said to be a chronic schizophrenic on drugs. A sheriff's deputy who knew him stated that he frequently stopped taking his prescribed drugs and then "became more crazy." A physical examination showed a thick green material coating his teeth. His chest was thought to be clear. The initial impression was acute schizophrenia.

A second examiner was then asked to see the patient. He noted that the patient's skin was very warm, and a repeat temperature was taken. Because the patient could not keep his mouth closed on the thermometer, a rectal temperature was obtained and it was 39.9°C. The patient was noted to be tachypneic with a respiratory rate of 36. A more careful chest exam now showed rales, bronchial breath sounds, and dullness over the left lower lung field. The patient appeared terrified and kept looking over his shoulder "for the five men who were after him to gun him down as they had shot his three friends last week." The police could be sure that such a mass murder hadn't taken place. Although this material was clearly delusional, he otherwise made sense and expressed his fears clearly.

A chest x-ray showed a left lower lobe pneumonia. Subsequent calls to the patient's wife revealed that he had been drinking heavily until three days earlier. The patient was admitted to the hospital and placed on high-dosage parenteral penicillin and sedation. He had a tumultuous early course, with delirium, and then slow partial clearing of his pneumonia. However, an effusion persisted, and eventually he required surgical decortication of the left lower lobe.

How can you differentiate an acute organic brain syndrome from schizophrenia?

What is the differential diagnosis in a "confused" patient?

In this patient the temperature was the secret, and the first reading taken was erroneous. One must feel the patient and judge the approximate temperature. If the estimate is not close to the recorded value, retake the temperature and be careful to exclude artifactual errors such as mouth breathing or sureptitious heating of the thermometer by the patient. In the emergency room it is repeatedly made clear that the key to appreciation of the presence of severe disease lies in accurately reading vital signs. This patient represents an acute toxic delirium and needs admission for intensive medical therapy.

Acute encephalopathy — usually metabolic rather than due to a mass lesion — can mimic a functional psychotic state fairly closely. We have seen intoxications with alcohol, scopolamine, amphetamines, lysergic acid (LSD), and others confused with functional psychosis. Hypoxia, hypotension, or hypoglycemia may present with features suggesting schizophrenia. Subarachnoid hemorrhage, meningitis, and encephalitis have been misconstrued as nonorganic psychosis. Steroid psychosis and collagen disease vasculitis may present in this way.

In general, the differential diagnosis of a "confused" patient includes three main groups: *confusion, dysphasia,* or *schizophrenia.*

The confused patient with a metabolic encephalopathy may have hallucinations, but these are usually visual (as opposed to the usually auditory ones in schizophrenia). The presence of a flap or ataxia argues for metabolic brain disease. Any abnormality of vital signs should lead to a search for metabolic or toxic causes of encephalopathy. Blood sugar, blood alcohol, arterial blood gas, and serum sodium analyses are appropriate in any confused patient. Paranoid ideation is common to any acute encephalopathy and in no way differentiates metabolic disorders from schizophrenia.

The presence of perseveration, gibberish speech, or anger with the frustration of expressive difficulties may reveal the presence of dysphasia. Often such a patient can pick the right information from a list even if he cannot spontaneously answer questions. The dysphasic or aphasic patient may be oriented, although it may not be initially apparent, and has no hallucinations or gross delusions.

The schizophrenic has been characterized as a cartoon character with an empty balloon over his head after he has finished talking. The listener cannot easily summarize what the patient just said. This is not usually true of the metabolic encephalopathy patient. Schizophrenics may make the physician feel amused or frightened or uncomfortable more than do encephalopathy patients.

A 52-YEAR-OLD MAN came to the emergency room. He was unable to give any symptoms and appeared obviously intoxicated. A brief physical exam revealed a strong odor of alcoholic beverages, blood pressure of 130/80, pulse of 84, temperature of 37.0°C, and respiratory rate of 20. He was ataxic. His speech was slurred. His blood alcohol level was 407 mg per 100 milliliters.

Twelve days earlier the man had come to the ER wishing "to donate my liver to the hospital." He had also been in the preceding day, one month earlier, and a total of twelve times in the past eighteen months. Usually he had no symptomatic complaints. Twice he had minor trauma problems. Several times he left before a physician could see him. He never wished to be put on any sort of program to avoid alcohol. His chart was 1 inch thick and consisted in only ER visit sheets plus occasional x-ray, lab, and ambulance reports.

After several hours in the ER, he appeared to be more sober and was referred to the social service staff for help in discontinuing his pattern of ER abuse.

What can the social service staff do for ER patients?

When should you involve them in a case?

41 DISCUSSION

Obviously, we have little to offer this patient. Perhaps one day he will be more interested in entering a detoxification unit and attempting to reduce his time on alcohol. At this time we can at least try to keep him from clogging the ER gears. The social service staff may be able to help. Appropriate referrals to Social Service include the following:

1. Patients whose psychological, social, or economic situation is interfering with medical treatment
   a. Patients who do not keep appointments, follow treatment, or take medications as prescribed
   b. Patients who use the emergency room inappropriately, i.e., those who come frequently yet have little wrong with them medically or who should be using other clinics
2. Counseling of families of patients
   a. Families in which a member is dying or has died
   b. Families who are anxious about the patient
   c. Families who are causing trouble for the medical staff or interfering with the treatment of the patient
   d. Suspected cases of child abuse. There might be situations where the doctor is not sure of the facts and the social worker might be able to clarify this by interviewing the parent(s). We also usually involve the pediatrics staff in such cases.
3. Patients who are experiencing social or economic problems as a result of physical or emotional illnesses
   a. Patients temporarily or permanently unable to work or who must change occupations
   b. Patients who can no longer continue a previous living arrangement
   c. Patients who are depressed over loss or need for adjustment caused by illness
   d. Patients who are experiencing adjustment problems in family relationships

4. Patients who in the opinion of medical personnel have emotional or social problems they are not adequately coping with and who might benefit from professional help. (This role clearly overlaps that of the ER psychiatry team, and either or both services may be used.)
   a. Depression, hostility, anxiety, disorientation, suspiciousness, dependency, self-destructiveness
   b. Need for legal aid or other specialized services
5. Patients needing placement in nursing homes or referral to other health programs

42

A 59-YEAR-OLD MAN was brought to the emergency room by ambulance. He had known chronic lung disease but had not been ill recently. This evening he was preparing for bed when his wife heard him gasp and fall over. She felt he was not breathing and called 911, the city emergency number. An ambulance quickly responded, and the patient was brought to the emergency room returning code 10-33 (red light and siren on). The ambulance attendant attempted to give cardiac massage and Ambu bag ventilation while en route.

The emergency room was notified of an incoming "arrest," and the resuscitation room was readied. The defibrillator paddles were coated with electrode jelly and one placed on the bed. One physician was detailed to ready tracheal intubation equipment. A second readied an Ambu bag and an oral airway. When the patient arrived, his chest was quickly stripped and he was thrown onto the bed. No pulse was palpable. He was given a shock of 400 watt seconds, then cardiac massage and bagging was begun. The ECG leads were attached and the monitor turned on. The rhythm was ventricular fibrillation. An intravenous route was established and $NaHCO_3$ (three ampules of 44 mEq each) was rapidly given. Another 400-watt-second shock was delivered, with no change. Bagging was attempted vigorously for fifteen seconds, and then the patient's trachea was intubated. Chest auscultation indicated both sides were being ventilated well. Cardiac massage was producing a palpable femoral pulse. The patient was given 1 mg of epinephrine by intracardiac needle via a xiphoid-costal angle puncture. Intracardiac blood was aspirated and then the epinephrine injected. He was given 10 ml of calcium chloride intravenously and two more ampules of bicarbonate. An arterial pH sample was drawn and the lab was asked to run it immediately; within two minutes the pH was reported to be 7.28. Two more ampules of bicarbonate were given. Lidocaine (100 mg) was given intravenously. Two more attempts at shock defibrillation were made.

Except for the brief times when a shock was being delivered, cardiac massage and ventilation were continued. The massage to ventilation ratio was held at 5:1. Despite these attempts, the patient's rhythm never changed from ventricular fibrillation. His pupils were initially dilated with no response to light, and stayed the same. After thirty minutes of resuscitation efforts the man was declared dead. Because intravenous lines had been inserted, he could not be called "Dead on Arrival" but was listed as "Probably Dead on Arrival, resuscitation unsuccessful."

Should you worry about giving an electrical shock to a pulseless patient without a diagnostic rhythm strip?

For optimal resuscitation, what should the ambulance crew have in equipment, personnel, and training?

What are the basic steps in cardiopulmonary resuscitation?

Most patients who suffer cardiac arrest are found to be in ventricular fibrillation when a rhythm can be determined. The chance of successfully defibrillating such a patient falls off rapidly with time. Early defibrillation is essential. There is indeed a hazard in shocking a patient who has no palpable pulse due to hypotension or supraventricular arrhythmias: The same ventricular fibrillation thought to be present initially may be brought about by the shock. Nonetheless, we would rather shock the pulseless patient first and look at the rhythm later.

An ambulance crew properly planned to handle emergency resuscitation would consist of at least three men. Most city ambulance services now use two-man teams. The crew would need skills in ventilation with Ambu bag and oral airway. They would need good cardiac massage technique and a van-type vehicle large enough to work over the patient on the trip. To function best, the crew would need skill in rhythm detection and a monitor defibrillator, perhaps with radio telemetry to the hospital. They would need intravenous infusion capabilities including sufficient height inside the vehicles to provide a pressure head for intravenous infusions. Probably drugs could be limited to $NaHCO_3$, atropine, lidocaine, and epinephrine. At this point most city or other ambulance services do not have these features satisfactorily covered, and ambulance resuscitation less often produces a good end result.

Once in the emergency room, a pulseless patient is resuscitated in a standardized fashion. Most importantly, one physician must take charge of the procedure. Seldom should any voice but his be heard, and he should not be involved directly in carrying out the procedures, but should observe and command the entire team. We suggest the following steps:

A. Attempt to reestablish spontaneous cardiac activity.
   1. Give blow to chest and wait fifteen seconds. If no pulse is felt:
   2. Defibrillate with 400-watt-second shock. If no pulse is felt, initiate cardiac massage.
B. Pulmonary-cardiac resuscitation (one physician assumes role of procedure chief).

1. Suction airway; place oral airway; bag with 100% O_2, keeping suction in place.
2. Massage started; continue massage in ratio 1:5.
3. Intubate trachea by cricothyroidotomy if necessary.
4. Evaluate effectiveness of ventilation and massage. The physician in charge must do this. If massage and ventilation are not being done correctly, no further steps are of any value.

C. Establish intravenous routes. Obtain physiologic parameters. Treat acidosis.
   1. Arm IV, large-bore, 2 ampules $NaHCO_3$
   2. CVP line (usually needed only later)
   3. Monitor and ECG: Defibrillate ventricular tachycardia or ventricular fibrillation immediately.
   4. Blood gas: Have lab called to do pH immediately.

D. Team coordinator evaluates data obtained and effectiveness of massage.

E. Attempts at definitive therapy: Continue massage and ventilation.
   1. Ventricular fibrillation
      a. Coarse fibrillation: direct current shock; lidocaine, 1 mg/kg/min to total of 5 mg/kg
      b. Fine fibrillation: intravenous or intracardiac epinephrine, 1 ml of 1/1000, or calcium gluconate or calcium chloride, 10 ml; direct current shock
      c. Recurrent refractory fibrillation: propanolol, 1 to 2 mg intravenously. Repeat in ten minutes if necessary.
   2. Asystole
      a. Intracardiac epinephrine, 1 mg; calcium gluconate or calcium chloride; direct current shock if fibrillation induced
      b. Pacemaker
   3. Electromechanical disassociation (electrical rhythm but no pulse)
      a. Isuprel, intravenously, 2 to 4 mg in 500 ml plus 1-mg bolus. Don't use if tachycardia or frequent VPCs present.
      b. Glucagon, 5 mg intravenously
      c. Calcium gluconate or calcium chloride, 10 ml intravenously
      d. Pressors: Aramine, 5 mg intravenously, or 100 to 200 mg per 500 ml drip. Levophed, 8 to 16 mg per 500 ml drip

      e. Mechanical assist.

      f. Consider pericardiocentesis.

4. AV block or bradycardia

      a. Atropine, 1 mg intravenously

      b. Isuprel, 2 to 4 mg per 500 ml drip

      c. Transvenous pacemaker

5. Acidosis

      a. One ampule of $NaHCO_3$ (44 mEq) every five minutes during arrest

      b. One bottle of $NaHCO_3$, 9% solution (500 ml has 300 mEq of $NaHCO_3$); run at 12 ml per minute or on a basis of blood gas.

6. Supraventricular tachyarrhythmia, atrial fibrillation, atrial flutter, paroxysmal atrial tachycardia, etc.

      a. Carotid massage, one side at a time

      b. Digoxin, .75 to 1 mg intravenously for fibrillation or flutter or PAT if not already on Digoxin

      c. Direct current shock if in cardiovascular collapse

      d. Propranolol, 1 mg intravenously

      e. Pressor trial; Neostigmine, 1 mg subcutaneously, or Tensilon, 10 mg slow IV push; remassage carotids.

43

A 59-YEAR-OLD MAN was brought to the emergency room by
ambulance. He complained of crushing chest pain for about one
hour. The pain had begun as he was riding in an elevator on the way
to work. He had become weak, dizzy, and sweaty. The pain radiated
to his mid upper back, but not his arms, neck, jaw, or elsewhere.
He was on no medications and had no prior medical problems.

On examination the patient was diaphoretic and writhing on the
bed. His blood pressure was 200/110, pulse 90 and regular. He had
no venous distention, a clear chest, no abnormalities of cardiac
impulse, and a faint S_3 gallop. He would hold his breath for several
seconds with pain several times a minute. The physician who saw
him believed he was suffering from a myocardial infarction, ordered
100 mg of Demerol, and went in search of a medical resident.

Before the Demerol was given, the patient stopped breathing and
had a seizure. Resuscitation was begun immediately, and he was
successfully returned to consciousness with respirations and a pulse.
Three days later he died in the coronary care unit with a sudden
ventricular rupture.

How do patients with symptomatic coronary artery disease
present in the ER?

Is it essential to make the diagnosis of myocardial infarction to
know you are dealing with a patient who might die suddenly?

Is there any ER therapy that could have been given that would
have prevented this patient's cardiac arrest in the ER?

There are two major problems facing the emergency-room physician who deals with patients with chest pain or other symptoms possibly due to coronary artery disease.

The first problem is the task of identifying which patients are likely to die suddenly. This is not entirely possible with available methods and is not synonymous with identifying patients who are suffering myocardial infarctions. Even the diagnosis of an acute myocardial infarction is not always easy. Frequently the patient does not present with a textbook description of crushing central chest pain associated with weakness, nausea, and diaphoresis. The patient may suffer a myocardial infarction and yet clearly deny chest pain. To approach this problem we suggest the following steps:

1. The history is the best source of data. Above all, do not invest too much security in the ECG. A normal ECG in no way precludes sudden death.
2. If a history of pain is not forthcoming, listen more for the circumstances surrounding the patient's decision to call for help. What was he doing and how did he feel? A patient who denies chest pain but says he felt that he was about to die probably had symptomatic coronary disease and should be admitted to the coronary care unit.
3. The physical examination must search for evidence of myocardial ischemia such as an enlarged apex beat, for evidence of congestive heart failure, and for arrhythmias. The pulse should be carefully felt throughout the interview.

The second task is that of preventing sudden death if possible. The patient needs rapid evaluation, rapid decision-making, and safe transportation from the ER to the coronary care unit. The most important initial therapy should be intravenous lidocaine (100 mg) if the pulse is over 70 and atropine (1 mg) if under 70. No time should be lost in the x-ray unit, and if possible a portable monitor defibrillator should accompany the patient to the coronary care unit. It is possible that this patient would not have had an arrest if treated with lidocaine quickly, since most cardiac arrests early in a myocardial infarction are due to ventricular arrhythmias. More than Demerol or a medical resident he needed to be on a monitor and to receive appropriate prophylactic antiarrhythmia therapy.

44

A 22-YEAR-OLD WOMAN came to the emergency room requesting a blood test. She planned to get married within one month. She was well and did not want to talk to a physician. Her encounter was handled entirely by a nurse. Blood samples were drawn for VDRL, blood type including Rh, and antirubella antibody titer. The lab results were to be sent to the gynecology clinic. The patient was told that she would there be seen by a physician, that a pelvic examination would probably be done, and that she could receive information about birth control if she wished. Nonetheless, the results were returned to the ER, and the patient came there for them. The VDRL was negative, blood type A, Rh positive, and rubella titer 1:80.

What should the patient be told?

The Colorado state law requires that a patient be examined and found free of venereal disease prior to marriage. Obviously, a negative VDRL argues against syphilis but in no way helps rule out other venereal diseases, especially the omnipresent gonorrhea. Law or no law, the physician should capitalize on this opportunity to do a pelvic examination and a culture for gonococcus, obtain a Pap smear, and assist the patient with desired information regarding sexual practices, pregnancy, contraception, etc.

Specifically, aside from urging this patient to keep her gynecology clinic appointment, you should tell her that the blood test for syphilis is negative, that her blood type is not the sort to lead to Rh problems for any of her babies, and that the rubella titer suggests that she had German measles and will not get it during pregnancy.

Most antirubella titers we see fall into two groups — 1:10 or less and 1:80 or more. The former group can be assumed to have inadequate immunity and the latter group to have adequate antibody. Officially, we view any titer over 1:10 as adequate to prevent German measles.

Obviously, several questions have not yet been covered. Among these is the possibility that the patient is already pregnant.

45

A 20-YEAR-OLD WOMAN came to the emergency room complaining of abdominal pain. She had been well previously and two days earlier had noted the onset of bilateral abdominal pain, most severe in the right lower abdomen, accompanied by nausea and vomiting. She had had no bowel movements for the past two days. She had noted no fever or chills and specifically denied any recent venereal disease or vaginal discharge. She was having sexual contacts and was on birth control pills. There was no prior history of abdominal or pelvic disease, and she had not had an appendectomy. Her last menstrual period had terminated three days earlier.

On physical examination, the patient appeared to be a young, healthy woman, who would pull away from an examining hand. Her blood pressure was 140/80, pulse 100, respiration 18, and temperature 38.0°C orally. The findings were normal except for her abdomen and pelvis. The abdomen was slightly distended, and she guarded throughout, especially the lower quadrants. Bowel sounds were present and unremarkable. The cervix was very tender, as were the uterus and adnexa. Because of this tenderness the adnexa could not be clearly palpated. A rectal examination demonstrated the tenderness to be largely anterior to the examining finger. Stool was brown and negative for occult blood.

What is the diagnosis?

How should the patient be treated?

What are the most common misdiagnoses made in a case such as this?

This woman probably has acute pelvic inflammatory disease (PID) — i.e., acute gonococcal salpingitis. She has been carrying the gonococcus indolently in her cervical canal for weeks, months, or even years. It is not clear what triggers the flare into an acute salpingitis, but this usually occurs just following a menstrual period. Differentiation from appendicitis is not always easy and relies on a careful physical exam with pelvic and rectal examinations. Occasionally a patient with PID is explored with a presumptive diagnosis of appendicitis. The recommended treatment is hospitalization with high-dose anti-biotics — usually penicillin intravenously. When this is impossible because of bed shortages or patient unwillingness, we have often been successful with outpatient therapy. We have been using 4.8 million units of procaine penicillin G and 1 gm of probenecid orally followed by oral doxycycline (Vibramycin), 100 mg bid for ten days. The patient must be seen the next day if not better and again in one week whether better or worse. There is a danger of tubo-ovarian abscesses and of tubal stenosis resulting in sterility. All the signs of an acute abdomen with peritonitis might develop in the patient, and, if so, clearly she would need hospitalization at that time. This patient is relatively nontoxic, and we could probably do well with her as an outpatient. Pelvic rest (no intercourse or douching) must be ad-hered to.

In general, the diagnostic problem in this sort of patient is dis-tinguishing between acute PID (or other acute pelvic visceral disasters, such as ruptured tubal pregnancy), appendicitis, and gastroenteritis. Perhaps the most helpful differential hint is that gastroenteritis does not begin with pain. It will begin with nausea, vomiting, diarrhea, anorexia, hydrogen sulfide eructation, etc., but seldom with pain. Pain, if it appears, comes later. On the other hand, appendicitis or PID almost invariably begins with pain. One must press the patient for the earliest symptoms. The pain of appendicitis usually begins periumbilically and moves to the right lower quadrant (RLQ) but may begin in the RLQ and stay there. Tenderness in appendicitis (on rectal or pelvic examination) is usually unilateral, whereas tenderness in PID is usually bilateral.

46

A 25-YEAR-OLD MAN came to the emergency room complaining of nausea and fatigue for two weeks. He claimed excellent health in the past and was working as a construction worker. Recently he found that he could barely make it through the day and several days missed work because of his fatigue. He admitted to smoking about one pack of cigarettes daily but denied more than an occasional alcoholic beverage. He was on no drugs but admitted "doing dope" in the past. He had been doing heroin and "speed" but had been straight for two months.

On physical examination the patient was observed to be a husky man in no apparent distress. Vital signs were normal. He was not jaundiced. His chest was clear, cardiovascular function normal, and he had no lymphadenopathy. There was right upper quadrant tenderness, and his liver seemed enlarged. In the midclavicular line the lower edge of the liver was palpable 15 cm below the percussible upper margin. He had a fullness of the left upper quadrant that was thought to be probably an enlarged spleen.

What is wrong with this patient?

How should he be handled?

Should his relatives be given gamma globulin?

This patient probably has hepatitis and probably has the long-incubation or serum hepatitis type. He is not clinically icteric but may still have an elevated serum bilirubin. Most observers cannot detect jaundice until the total bilirubin is over 2 mg per 100 milliliters. However, the urine may contain enough conjugated bilirubin ("direct-reacting bilirubin") to display yellow foam if shaken or to produce a positive ictotest.

Hepatitis when seen in our ER is usually of viral or toxic etiology. The virus may be short-incubation "infectious hepatitis" with an incubation period of two to six weeks and no Australia antigen (hepatitis-associated antigen, HAA) present. It may be parenterally transmitted long-incubation (six to twenty-four weeks) "serum hepatitis" with HAA present at some time during the course. (Probably HAA is no longer present in this case.) Hepatitis may be due to mononucleosis, indicated by a positive mono spot test and heterophil antibody titer. Viral hepatitis usually presents with a prodrome of several weeks of malaise, anorexia, and miscellaneous functional-sounding symptoms. A rash or arthralgias may begin the illness.

Toxins producing hepatitis include many chemicals and drugs. Antituberculosis therapy, halothane anesthesia, and others have been incriminated. In our ER the most common hepatotoxin is ethyl alcohol. Alcoholic hepatitis seems to act as a bridge between fatty liver and cirrhosis.

We usually obtain a weight on our presumed hepatitis patient. Anorexia or vomiting severe enough to cause continual weight loss may eventually lead to hospitalization. One should document this with serial weight measurements. We draw biochemical survey, CBC, prothrombin time, HAA, and bilirubin (direct and indirect); and we obtain a urinalysis or a chest x-ray if findings suggest these. We would refer this patient to a weekly hepatitis clinic in our hospital. By that time his lab data will be available.

Close contacts of patients with infectious hepatitis (IH; short-incubation, nonparenteral transmission) should receive gamma globulin as soon as possible to lessen the severity of the disease if they contract it. We use the immunization clinic in the Disease Control branch of the local Department of Public Health for dispensing gamma globulin. To dispense it they need an official report of the defined case. Any patient with presumed IH should be reported to Disease Control by filling out the appropriate form. Contacts of serum hepatitis (SH) patients, on the other hand, have far less chance of contracting SH by an oral route. In addition, the gamma globulin available has a low titer of antibody against SH and may be useless. Usually it is not recommended in such a case. Occasionally it is given (in a low dose — 0.02 ml per pound of body weight up to 2.0 ml maximum dose), especially when the diagnosis of SH is unclear.

A 40-YEAR-OLD MAN came to the emergency room because he needed a refill of his prescriptions. He was a known seizure patient who was taking phenobarbital, 32 mg orally qid, and diphenyl-hydantoin (Dilantin), 100 mg orally tid. On this regimen he had had no seizures during the past six months. He had been out of town and had missed a scheduled neurology clinic appointment. Because of this his prescriptions had run out two days earlier. His next neurology clinic appointment was in three weeks; he had made this appointment today to replace the one he had missed. Today he had no complaints — he said he had never felt better.

The interviewing nurse obtained a set of vital signs, which were normal, and filled out two prescriptions. An intern observed the patient's gait, noted the absence of nystagmus, and signed the prescriptions and the encounter form.

What prescriptions should be refilled?

Can a nurse write a prescription legally?

We generally do not refill prescriptions in the ER or the receiving unit except those in the following categories and then only for the amount needed to last to the next appointment: (1) cardiac medications (digitalis, antiarrhythmics), (2) diuretics, (3) antihypertensive medications, (4) antiseizure medications, (5) diabetes drugs such as insulin, (6) phenothiazines for known schizophrenics. Pain medications are refillable at the discretion of the physician. In general, we do not refill prescriptions for chronic pain medications or chronic sedative or psychoactive drugs. We urge such patients to contact their primary physicians or to get medical clinic appointments.

Some patients who present with a request for a prescription refill really need anything but that. A patient may present with a request for a refill on a noneffective drug prescribed for the wrong reason for a misdiagnosed illness. His symptoms must be evaluated as with any other patient, and he needs a workup with appropriate therapy.

A nurse may fill out any of the information on a prescription form except the physician's signature. Office nurses for private practitioners often communicate refill orders to pharmacies. Indeed, as long as the prescription has been reviewed and signed by a physician, the bulk of it may be written by anyone in the unit.

A 56-YEAR-OLD MAN came to the emergency room complaining of chronic back pain for many years. He felt he was disabled and unable to work. He had been referred to the ER by the welfare department. He denied more than mild alcohol intake and smoked one pack of cigarettes daily. He denied other symptoms.

A brief physical examination showed normal gait, no muscle spasm in the lumbar paraspinal muscles, normal symmetric reflexes, and normal vital signs. The patient was referred to the orthopedic clinic for further evaluation.

What is a "welfare patient"?

Some patients who are on welfare (disabled, dependent children, or other) arrive at the emergency room with symptoms. They are treated as any other patient would be except that they usually are financially covered by Medicaid and a different prescription blank is used.

However, in our ER the term *welfare patient* has come to mean the patient who wishes to get on welfare and has some medical problem that is disabling to him. These patients often first go to the welfare department because they have run out of money, lost their lodging, or just arrived in town. If they claim medical disability as cause for needing welfare assistance, they are referred to the ER.

We should in a preliminary check try to determine the degree of acuteness of the disabling problem. If it appears fairly acute, we examine fully and evaluate the patient. Then the diagnosis and estimate of duration of disability are noted on an Assistance Clearance and Registration form. The ER social worker then arranges for temporary assistance to the patient.

If the disabling problem is chronic and seems not to be acutely changed, we usually do not do an evaluation in the ER. This works a hardship for the patient, since there may be a six-week delay, but the ER cannot cope with the demand otherwise. We refer the patient to the appropriate clinic (medical, surgical, orthopedics, etc.) and to the welfare department if he has not already been there. Eventually, when the workup is complete, the patient will be seen in the Aid to Needy and Dependent (AND) clinic, which will evaluate the final workup.

A 26-YEAR-OLD MAN walked into the emergency room requesting a brief physical examination for a chauffeur's license. He was applying for a job as an ambulance driver with a private company nearby. He stated that he was well and that he had already passed the eye exam for his license. The physician was not sure what constituted an appropriate physical examination in this context but began by taking the patient's blood pressure. The pressure was 200/140 in the right arm, seated or supine, and about the same in the left arm. The pedal pulses were palpable with a blood pressure cuff around the lower thigh inflated to 220 mm Hg. Both eyes had narrow arteriolar segments, AV nicking, and many areas of hemorrhage and exudate in the fundi. The optic discs were flat and distinct. The rest of the physical findings were normal.

The patient was surprised to be told that he had high blood pressure. He did not want to be admitted to the hospital but agreed to allow appropriate studies to be done and to return to the medical clinic in two days for initiation of therapy. An electrocardiogram, posterior-anterior (P-A) and lateral chest x-rays, and CBC, electrolyte, BUN, glucose, and creatinine analyses were done. The examining physician arranged for the patient to be seen two days later by a physician friend in the second physician's medical clinic. The next available appointment in our medical clinic was three weeks off, and that seemed too far in the future.

The patient did not keep his appointment two days later and instead went on an eight-week vacation to his parents' home 1500 miles away. He returned to the ER two months after his first visit, confused, complaining of headaches, and with papilledema. At that time his blood pressure was 240/160. He was admitted to the hospital and treated for malignant or accelerated hypertension. His creatinine clearance at this time was 20 ml per minute.

What might have tipped off the physician at the first visit that this patient might not be as reliable as he seemed?

When is hypertension an emergency?

Hypertension is usually not viewed as an emergency itself unless it has entered into the accelerated phase. This phase consists of rapidly progressing damage to small vessels with development of encephalopathy, rapid decline of renal function, and optic fundal changes of hemorrhages, exudates, or papilledema. This patient had a severe elevation of his diastolic pressure and optic changes of grade-3 hypertensive retinopathy. It might have been expected that his thinking was affected and that he might make unwise decisions. His decision not to keep his appointment should have been anticipated. This patient should have been vigorously urged to accept hospitalization on his first visit to the ER. Failing that, therapy should have been begun at that time.

Long-standing diastolic hypertension does increase the likelihood of a stroke or a myocardial infarction. It is difficult to refrain from becoming anxious when your patient has a diastolic pressure of 120 to 150 mm Hg even if it is of long standing. In the absence of signs of severe retinopathy, nephropathy, or encephalopathy, however, we usually defer initiating treatment in the ER.

One remarkable feature of this case was the fact that the patient was seen by a physician at all on his first visit to the ER. Non-emergency physical examinations for well patients are not done in the ER. Only the physician's sympathy for this man, who had waited over two hours at that time, led him to do the examination.

50

A 56-YEAR-OLD MAN came to the ER complaining of pain in his right thigh. He had bumped it getting out of a car two days earlier, and it was getting more painful and swollen. Because his regular physician was out of town, he came to the ER. He had suffered a myocardial infarction six months earlier and was still on coumarin anticoagulant for this.

On examination, a large blue bruise covering the anterior lower right thigh was observed. A sample was drawn to check prothrombin time, and the patient was sent for an x-ray of the thigh. The x-ray was normal. By the time the patient returned from the radiology department, the physician caring for him had finished his twelve-hour shift and signed his cases over to another physician. The second physician noted that the x-ray pictures were normal and discharged the patient. The patient, however, was unsatisfied and went to another emergency room, where he was hospitalized. We later noted the prothrombin time to be 45 seconds with a control of 11 seconds.

Was this an example of a physician's error, a patient's error, or a failure of the medical system?

How should the patient have been treated?

What instructions should patients be given when they are placed on anticoagulant therapy?

This patient was handled correctly initially, but there was a lapse in care in the change of physicians. Obviously, if a laboratory test is worth doing, the results should be obtained and acted on. Not infrequently a patient is signed over to another physician at a shift change and the new physician fails to review the course of events properly and take over management of the problems being presented.

One must wonder why this patient did not question the second physician about the prothrombin time. He obviously was unsatisfied, but he did not communicate his dissatisfaction to the physician. Was this primarily a failure on the patient's part, a failure of the lab to provide data rapidly enough, or the physician's failure? Probably all three. Nonetheless, the physician must be assumed to have the ultimate responsibility.

Proper therapy for this patient would include bed rest, withdrawal of the anticoagulant, and probably some vitamin K to allow synthesis of needed clotting factors by the liver. Vitamin K is fat soluble and needs bile salts for absorption. If there is any suggestion of obstructive liver disease (intrahepatic or extrahepatic), the vitamin K should be given parenterally. To avoid another hematoma it is usually given intravenously rather than intramuscularly in a 5- to 10-mg dose. Oral therapy is often acceptable. "Rebound hypercoagulability," an often stated danger, probably is not as hazardous as over-anticoagulation.

Therapeutic anticoagulation with drugs related to coumarin is usually monitored with the quick prothrombin time. The prothrombin time is usually kept between 2 and 2½ times the control. In any case, bleeding while on coumarin must be recognized as a dangerous problem. The patient must know that he should discontinue use of the anticoagulant and see his physician. He should also know that many other drugs are dangerous when one is on coumarin and that over-the-counter preparations should not be taken without checking with his physician. Most important, he should remind his physician when seeing him that he is on an anticoagulant. Patients usually assume their physicians remember everything, a dangerous assumption.

51

AN 80-YEAR-OLD MAN was sent to the ER by ambulance from a nursing home because "his catheter was plugged." On arrival he seemed confused and could not give any useful history. His Foley catheter was indeed plugged and could not be irrigated. Vital signs were obtained, and they were normal. A new bladder catheter was easily placed to replace the old one. It immediately drained 700 ml of slightly cloudy urine and subsequently drained 100 ml over the next two hours. He was returned to the nursing home.

What usually causes anuria?

Are there any dangers in relieving lower urinary tract obstruction in this fashion?

What other urologic emergencies may be seen in the ER?

Anuria usually is due to an obstruction. Oliguria usually is not. Acute glomerulonephritis (especially in children) and cortical necrosis due to drugs or hypoxia can present with anuria, but generally anuria means obstruction, and this is only rarely due to bilateral upper urinary tract obstruction unless the patient has only one functioning kidney due to prior trauma, surgery, or disease. In general, the anuric patient will be found with distended bladder and an inability to void. Acute overdistention may occur in a beer-drinker who won't urinate. A history of prostatism (nocturia, post-voiding dribbling, slow stream, etc.) is usually present. Acute voiding inability usually responds to a single catheterization.

The patient with a chronic obstruction who has overflow incontinence needs relief of obstruction with catheterization or suprapubic aspiration. Rapid decompression (over 100 ml per hour) may be dangerous; it may result in a glomerular diuresis of great volume, and the patient may go into shock due to loss of fluid and electrolytes. This is rare, but the patient should be observed for several hours. If he is passing urine at a rate of over 200 ml per hour or his blood pressure is dropping, he should be returned to the ER, probably for hospital admission and vigorous fluid repletion.

Other urologic emergencies seen in the ER include trauma, torsion of the testis, colic, septicemia, priapism, hematuria, a scrotal mass, and in a child an abdominal mass.

52

A 38-YEAR-OLD WOMAN was taken to another hospital's emergency room by concerned relatives. She stated that she awoke in the morning and saw two strange men in her house. She called the police, but the men mysteriously disappeared. Later there were "several zebras walking across the wall." Her son stated that she was a heavy drinker and that she drank to keep from being nervous.

On physical examination the patient was noted to have a tachycardia (120) but to be afebrile. Her blood pressure was 114/90. She was anxious and tachypneic but well oriented. Reflexes were brisk and pupils dilated but reactive. She complained of thirst and a dry mouth. She was given 100 mg of Librium intramuscularly. A resident was called to see her. He noted a peripheral neuropathy. His diagnoses were: (1) DTs, (2) alcoholic myopathy and neuropathy, and (3) depression. She was referred to our ER for admission to the alcohol detoxification unit.

On arrival at our ER the woman denied much recent drinking. Her blood pressure was 100/70 supine and 80/65 sitting, and her pulse was 120 sitting. A hematocrit was 42% and stool hematest negative. She said she really didn't want to go to the detoxification ward — she didn't consider herself to be an alcoholic. The staff physician seeing her pointed out that not everyone in the ER that day was hallucinating, and the sooner she realized she was an alcoholic the sooner she might be able to do something about it.

Samples were drawn for CBC, electrolytes, BUN, sugar, biochemical survey, VDRL, and blood alcohol analyses; and urinalysis and chest x-rays were done. The patient was admitted to the alcohol detoxification unit, and ten minutes later the electrolytes were reported to be: Na 118, Cl 83, HCO_3 9, and K 2.8 mEq/L. Alcohol level was only 27 mg per 100 milliliters. A phone call to the woman's relatives uncovered the fact that she had indeed

been depressed and probably had taken an overdose of aspirin and
Sleep-eez, an over-the-counter sedative containing scopolamine.
Serum salicylate level was 47 mg per 100 milliliters.

Did the patient have DTs?

Why was she hallucinating?

How do you treat overdoses of acetylsalicylic acid (aspirin)?

Would it be a good idea for the woman to recognize the fact that
she is an alcoholic?

52 DISCUSSION

Although this patient is indeed an alcoholic, she probably was not hallucinating due to alcohol withdrawal. She clearly does not have DTs; she is neither delirious nor tremulous. Scopolamine is one of the more common hallucinogens, and over-the-counter sedative overdoses often present with hallucinations. We usually treat such a patient with physostigmine, 2 mg subcutaneously or intravenously as often as every thirty minutes. This patient might have benefited from such therapy earlier. Her dry mouth and dilated pupils might have been warning signs of the responsible agent. Other drugs such as bromides or lysergic acid (LSD) may also cause hallucinations.

Salicylate toxicity is often underestimated. The patient is usually awake and alert, so the usual worrisome signs of coma are not available to orient the physician. Serious salicylate overdoses usually present with serum levels over 80 mg per 100 milliliters. We generally don't worry when patients have levels under 60 mg per 100 milliliters. If we do treat, it usually is with forced alkaline diuresis. We use a solution of 1000 ml D5/0.2 normal saline plus 44 mEq $NaHCO_3$ plus 20 mEq KCl, and infuse it at 2000 ml per hour. This can produce pulmonary edema, so the patient must be watched carefully with chest x-rays, intake and output records, and chest auscultation. Since this can derange sodium or potassium levels and can produce dangerous levels of alkalosis, these parameters must be carefully monitored. Most of these patients need admission, especially if the salicylate level is over 80 mg per 100 milliliters.

In the end, alcoholism will be the patient's major problem. However, correction of her present metabolic abnormalities must precede any significant psychiatric therapy. She shouldn't be obliged to admit to being an alcoholic to get such therapy. Alcoholism does not limit the patient's susceptibility to other drugs or diseases, but it often leads the physician away from a careful consideration of other diagnoses.

A 45-YEAR-OLD MAN was brought to the ER by ambulance. He was said to have ingested several drugs. On arrival he was drowsy but arousable. Although he refused to communicate, he could walk and had a good gag reflex. He was given syrup of ipecac, 30 ml orally, and 300 ml of warm tap water. This resulted in copious vomiting over the next thirty minutes. The patient was kept in the emergency room and observed. After three hours he seemed more alert and was walking about and asking the staff for cigarettes. He was referred to the ER psychiatry team for further evaluation. Perusal of his old chart revealed that he had long carried the diagnosis of paranoid schizophrenia and had been on phenothiazines in the past.

The nurse on the psychiatry team saw the patient in the fifth hour of his ER stay and reported to the referring physician that he was too sleepy to interview. On rechecking he was found to be comatose and unresponsive to pain but breathing well and with a normal blood pressure. His pockets were emptied and found to contain prescription bottles for Thorazine, Seconal, and Kemadrin. A nasotracheal tube was easily placed, his stomach was lavaged with 2 liters of tap water via a Ewald tube, and he was admitted to the medical intensive care unit.

Why do overdose patients have fluctuating levels of consciousness?

What is "observation" in the ER?

This patient probably took more of his drugs covertly after entering the ER. He was a "double overdose." We occasionally observe an alcoholic becoming more drunk during his stay in the ER (more ataxic, sleepier, thicker speech) and find a half-full bottle of wine in his clothing. Usually overdose patients are stripped and searched and thus relieved of any drugs.

Varying depth of coma may be due to:

1. On and off GI absorption. This is true for any drug but classic for meprobamate, which forms concretions in the gut. Duodenal storage may have been the problem here, and a cathartic should have been given.
2. Enterohepatic circulation
3. Secondary effect of hypoxia on consciousness
4. Brief action of narcotic antagonists versus long action of opiates
5. Brief action of glucose versus long-acting hypoglycemic agents
6. Subdural hematomas (especially worrisome in an alcoholic who is not properly waking up)
7. Repeated ingestion, as in this case

Certain words have awesome implications in our ER that are not conveyed by their literal meaning. *Observed* should mean closely watched, yet often it is used to mean patient neglected, booth curtain closed, and no further evaluation. *Stable* is another such term. It should mean at least two successive observations the same with time intervening. Yet often we use it when we mean one set of normal vital signs with no temporal observations at all.

A 28-YEAR-OLD POLICEMAN was brought to the ER by ambulance. He had made a call on a residence to investigate a prowler complaint. After an initial inspection he knocked on the house door. The occupant reached around the partly opened door and fired a revolver at the policeman. Once the deed was done, he looked at his victim and called for an ambulance.

On arrival at the ER the patient was alive. He had a pulse and obtainable blood pressure of 140/80. His respirations were spontaneous at a rate of 14. He had an entrance wound between the eyebrows and an exit wound posteriorly just to the right of the occiput. His pupils were midposition and reactive. He was comatose with no response to voice or painful stimuli.

An endotracheal tube was placed, and the patient was hyperventilated with an Ambu bag at a rate of 30 per minute. Two intravenous routes were started and a solution of 5% dextrose in water was run very slowly at a keep-open rate. He was given 50 gm of Mannitol and 10 mg of dexamethasone intravenously. In the operating room an anterior craniotomy was done. The damaged right frontal lobe was debrided, the frontal sinus lining was curetted, and the craniotomy was closed. A similar procedure was done posteriorly. Two weeks later the patient left the hospital with a left hemiparesis.

How predictable is the outcome of head injury?

What is the reason for the hyperventilation, Mannitol, and steroid therapy?

The results of head injuries are not always predictable. One should not hesitate to treat patients with even disastrous-appearing injuries.

In general, an anterior-posterior (A-P) bullet course is more likely to be benign than a side-to-side wound. Nonetheless, many bullets take courses not defined by a straight line connecting entrance and exit wounds. A high-velocity bullet tends to take a straighter course than a low-velocity missile.

Initial therapy includes attempts at avoiding brain edema. "Brain shrinkage" is best accomplished with a 100- to 300-gm intravenous bolus of Mannitol (2 to 3 gm/kg), dexamethasone (10 mg initially and 4 mg every six hours thereafter), and hyperventilation, which is probably the most effective maneuver. Neurosurgical therapy must be prompt even though the brain is already partly decompressed by the bullet wound of the cranium.

A 20-YEAR-OLD MAN walked into the ER. He told the interviewing nurse that he had been in an auto accident three hours earlier but had felt more or less all right and had gone home. Then his shoulders, arms, and neck began to hurt, so his mother told him to go to the hospital. When he arrived, he was placed in the main ER, where he was interviewed by one of the more junior physicians available.

A full examination was done, including full range of movement of the neck. Then a complete set of cervical spine films was obtained, including flexion, extension, and odontoid views. The radiologist was not available, so the physician viewed the films alone. He mentioned to a staff physician that he had an interesting case of cervical spondylolisthesis. The second physician immediately placed sandbags on either side of the patient's head and a cervical collar on his neck. He told the patient not to move his head. A review of the films indeed disclosed an unstable cervical fracture-dislocation of C5-6. Skull tongs were placed, and the patient was admitted to the hospital for constant traction.

What is the usual presentation of a broken neck?

How should it be cared for in the emergency room?

What is the danger to the patient of further neck movement?

What particular sporting injury should always suggest cervical fractures?

This patient had no apparent neurologic defect. By amazing luck his injury had not yet impinged on his cervical cord or nerve roots. The most common spinal fracture site is at the C6-7 vertebral level, which impinges on the cord structures at the T1 neurologic level. The patient usually is brought in by stretcher with his arms flexed at the elbow and his hands together on his chest. He has flaccid paralysis elsewhere and may have hypotension due to loss of sympathetic innervation. If the day is hot, his temperature may be elevated due to absence of sweating.

One should sandbag the patient's head straight. If it is turned, we usually try to straighten it gently with traction. If he is alert, he must be told to hold his head perfectly still, and if not, someone must constantly hold his head in place. This patient cannot be left alone. A cross-table lateral x-ray of the cervical spine should be done first. His arms should be pulled slowly down toward his feet before the x-ray — otherwise spasm of the shoulders will obscure much of the film below C5. The x-ray should be carefully inspected for misalignment of the posterior border of the vertebral bodies. If a fracture seems present, only an A-P film should then be taken and the patient immobilized by skeletal traction on the same stretcher with only one move of the patient — onto a circle bed or frame after placement of tong traction.

Any movement may render the patient paraplegic or quadraplegic (depending on the injury level). If quadraplegia develops and is still present after twenty-four hours of traction, there is little chance of any recovery.

There are two common types of incomplete cord injuries:

1. Loss of all but position and vibratory senses. The injury occurs (as do most spine injuries) with neck flexed. Probably the anterior spinal artery is damaged, whereas the two smaller posterior spinal arteries are less badly damaged. These cases may recover well if incomplete injury occurs.
2. Posterior cord injury with loss of central crossing fibers. The patient may have flaccid paralysis of arms and fairly normal legs. The prognosis is usually good.

Trampoline accidents are especially likely to fracture the cervical spine, and in any such patient a spine fracture should be suspected. Head injury is often associated with neck injury, and we should probably be taking many more cervical x-rays (and probably fewer skull series) than we do. Pain or tenderness over the spinous processes, as opposed to the large neck muscles, suggests the presence of a fracture. A full range of motion exam should not be done on such a patient nor should a full set of cervical x-ray views be obtained.

56

A 48-YEAR-OLD WOMAN came to the ER claiming that she had been in a fight with her husband. She smelled of alcohol, was disheveled, and lapsed into tears periodically. She had multiple puffy, bruised areas about her face, and her nose was obviously crooked. Both eyes were puffy, and one was almost shut. She was breathing easily and had normal vital signs. The resident radiologist recommended sinus views and a nasal view. The only abnormality of the bones was a fractured nose. She was sent home with an ice pack and told to return the next day to the ear-nose-throat (ENT) clinic to have her nose adjusted.

How do you determine what is broken in facial trauma?

What x-ray views may be helpful?

The first concerns in facial trauma have to do with airway and neck and brain injuries. Laryngeal trauma can accompany facial trauma, and laryngeal edema may be progressive. Once these are dealt with, the bones of the face should be carefully palpated. Both sides must be compared at each step. Palpate the zygomatic arch, the orbital rim, and the jaw. Anesthesia of the infraorbital nerve suggests a fracture. The most important question to ask a patient with a suspected mandibular or maxillary fracture is whether his teeth fit together properly.

Midface fractures may be maxillary — usually occurring in major trauma such as those sustained in auto accidents. They may be blowout fractures of the orbit with an intact orbital rim and orbital floor collapse. They may be tripod fractures of the zygomatic arch, or they may be nasal fractures. There may be cerebrospinal rhinorrhea and associated basal skull fractures. Of all these, the nasal fracture is most common and most benign. We usually do no emergency manipulation of a nasal fracture but let the swelling subside a bit.

Mandibular fractures may present with many loose foreign bodies (teeth, etc.) that can be aspirated by the patient if he is at all obtunded and lying on his back. There are often associated mouth wounds, making the fracture compound. In such cases we usually close all layers of the laceration and give the patient antibiotics.

There are many possible x-rays for facial fractures. We can get skull views, nasal films, mandibular films, orbital films, etc. In general, a sinus series is best. We frequently add mandibular views — P-A plus right and left oblique — and a Towne's view.

57

A 30-YEAR-OLD MAN was brought to the ER by ambulance after his family called the city emergency number 911, reported that he was bleeding seriously from a cut, and requested an ambulance. The policemen who arrived minutes before the ambulance found a husky man with a tourniquet on his left upper arm and a 4-cm wound laterally on his forearm. They replaced the tourniquet with a bath towel local pressure bandage. The ambulance attendant removed this and found a no-longer-bleeding wound, which he bound with a sterile dressing.

Before leaving the scene the ambulance attendant followed the trail of blood through the patient's house to the basement, where he noticed a small wooden table with a sharply broken leg. The table leg was splintered, and the attendant noted the possibility of splinters in the wound. He estimated there was about 500 ml of blood about the house.

On his arrival at the ER, the patient's wound was anesthetized, cleaned, and irrigated. A gloved finger could be inserted subcutaneously for about 8 centimeters.

How do lay people generally try to stop bleeding?

How would you treat this wound?

It is amazing how few people realize that pressure over a wound is appropriate to hold bleeding in check. We have people appearing at the ER who have tried to stop bleeding by applying anything from vitamin A to turpentine to the wound. Most people seem to be of the "dab and look" school, applying inadequate pressure for inadequate time and then checking to see if it is still bleeding. This patient probably lost a unit of blood, thanks in part to a tourniquet applied at too low a pressure.

The keystone of wound care is adequate debridement. All wounds are contaminated. Problems that arise almost always can be traced to ineffective removal of this contamination during initial treatment. Wounds are contaminated by damaged or dead tissues and by ground-in dirt and bacteria. Removal of dead or damaged tissue and ground-in dirt or bacteria will leave a wound that heals primarily, leaving a minimal scar. Removal of dead or damaged tissue is accomplished by sharp excision of obvious necrotic material and ragged subcutaneous tissue, with "freshening up" of skin edges. This can be done with fine (Iris) scissors or a scalpel. Removal of embedded. dirt or bacteria is accomplished by copiously irrigating the depths of the wound with a bulb syringe using at least 500 ml of saline solution for a moderate laceration (5 to 6 cm) and more for a larger laceration. This cannot be adequately done in a wound that has not been previously anesthetized.

This patient's wound was opened with a scalpel to the full extent of the undermined tunnel. Several splinters of wood were removed. The rough skin edges were debrided and the opened wound re-scrubbed and irrigated. It was then sutured closed. The wound was closed in two steps. The subcutaneous tissues were closed with 3-0 chromic catgut and the skin with 4-0 Prolene. The patient was given tetanus toxoid and told to return to the surgical wound clinic in two days to have his wound reexamined.

58

A 77-YEAR-OLD WOMAN was brought to the ER complaining of constipation. She had had trouble with bowel function for over ten years and had been diagnosed as having Parkinson's disease for the past five years. At present she was on L-dopa and 1 teaspoonful of Metamucil daily. She complained of diffuse abdominal cramping pain, vomiting, and squirts of diarrhea despite a feeling of inability to pass a stool. On physical examination she had normal vital signs and a mildly tender abdomen. Her rectum was vastly distended by soft, brown stool that tested negative for occult blood.

The physician caring for her felt that she had obstipation resulting in a partial rectal obstruction.

Does Parkinson's disease lead to constipation?

How should the patient be treated?

Most patients with Parkinson's syndrome are old, and colonic malfunction is common in the old. Probably the neurologic disease itself does not lead to constipation, but of course, such patients are often treated with anticholinergics, and these drugs may induce more rectal dysfunction.

Therapy should begin with vigorous cleaning out of the distended rectum. This can usually be done with enemas. After they were unsuccessful in this patient she was given 10 mg of morphine subcutaneously. Nupercaine anesthetic ointment was placed in the anal canal, and the impaction was removed bit by bit digitally.

The woman was then allowed to rest for an hour and sent home with instructions to use a tap water enema once a day for three days; to drink at least 2 quarts of fluid daily; to take 2 teaspoonfuls of Metamucil in water four times daily followed each time by a glass of hot water. She was encouraged to take a large glass of prune juice each morning; not to ignore any urge for a bowel movement; and to set aside a time each morning after breakfast to attempt a bowel movement. She was told that if she went three days with no evacuation she should use glycerine suppositories, and, if that was unsuccessful, a tap water enema.

Since the diarrhea is a sort of overflow incontinence as a result of obstipation, opiates would be antitherapeutic and should not be used.

59

A 43-YEAR-OLD MAN came to the ER by ambulance. He said that he had swallowed half a hot dog and that it was stuck in his throat. He was anxious but otherwise seemed well. The physical examination turned up nothing remarkable. He was reassured and sent home.

The next morning, twelve hours later, he reappeared at the ER even more distressed. Now he was constantly drooling into a basin that he carried. He collected about 100 ml of saliva in two hours in the ER. An upper GI x-ray study showed an obstructing mass in the distal esophagus. This was removed bit by bit by esophagoscopy. It was indeed a hot dog.

How do you make the diagnosis of a partial esophageal obstruction?

What is a café coronary?

Was this one?

Esophageal obstruction commonly presents in this way, and typically no one believes the patient who says he has an esophageal obstruction. Meat impaction is common even without the presence of organic disease of the distal esophagus. There is much discomfort and a serious potential of emesis with aspiration. The patient should be taken seriously and treated quickly. If the patient is seen after about one hour, he is usually drooling copious quantities of saliva. He often sits quietly with his head bowed over a towel or basin and can be diagnosed from across the room. We do not advise the use of enzymes or meat tenderizer; these agents are very irritating and destructive to an already damaged esophageal mucosa. The patient needs endoscopy, which is usually done with local anesthesia at any time of the day or night.

A "café coronary" refers to the sudden death of a restaurant patron choking on a large piece of food. This is usually steak in a patient who usually has consumed several alcoholic beverages. The patient may have dentures or may be a voluble talker while eating. The food lodges in the hypopharynx and pushes the trachea closed or obstructs in the glottis. Treatment must be immediate or all is lost. Café coronary patients do not make it to the ER. The food should be removed digitally, and if this doesn't clear an airway, a stab wound cricothyroidotomy should be done. Despite the name, the coronary arteries are not implicated in this illness.

60

A 33-YEAR-OLD WOMAN was brought to the ER by ambulance. She had passed out at home and then awoke with several concerned relatives in attendance. She felt weak and experienced bouts of uncontrollable shivering. The ambulance was called by dialing 911, the all-purpose city emergency number, and she was brought to the ER. On arrival she admitted to a week's illness with malaise and myalgias, rhinorrhea, and nonproductive cough. She had diagnosed herself as suffering from "the flu" and had called her physician, who did not see her but sent out a prescription for ampicillin. She took one 250-mg capsule and within thirty minutes had lost consciousness. The rest of her history was not helpful.

The initial physical examination showed a temperature of 36.0°C rectally, pulse thready at 60, blood pressure unobtainable, and respiratory rate 18. The patient was very alert and well oriented and in no way obtunded. Her chest was clear and heart tones faint but otherwise normal. Her skin was pale with a noticeable pallor of the lips, but there was a faint pink hue to the abdominal skin. A brief neurologic examination showed no gross abnormalities, and her abdomen was benign. The rectal exam was normal, with brown stool that was negative when tested for occult blood.

The initial diagnosis was shock of unknown etiology. The patient's ECG showed diffuse ST segment depression, thought to be ischemic. Nasal oxygen was placed and begun at a flow rate of 5 liters per minute. Two large intravenous routes were placed and 1000 ml of normal saline solution was given in thirty minutes. At this point a central venous pressure reading of 3 cm of saline was obtained, and systolic blood pressure became audible at 60 mm Hg. The patient was given 0.3 mg of epinephrine (0.3 ml of 1:1000 solution) subcutaneously with no obvious results, and then 0.3 mg intravenously. At this point she complained of excruciating pain in her head, chest, back, and abdomen which lasted over five minutes. Her systolic blood pressure rose to 90 and then returned to 60. Because of her relative bradycardia (rate 60) and the unusual response to epinephrine, she was given 1.0 mg of atropine intravenously. This doubled her cardiac rate and brought her blood pressure briefly to 120/70 but she again had severe pain, this time lasting ten minutes.

Drug therapy was discarded, and the patient was given more saline. Within two hours of her arrival in the ER she had been given 4000 ml of saline and had a systolic pressure of 80 mm Hg. She was admitted to the intensive care unit with a diagnosis of anaphylactic shock. A portable chest x-ray had been normal, and arterial blood gas levels were unremarkable except for a pH of 7.34 due to a mild metabolic acidosis. She improved steadily over the next twelve hours, no further laboratory abnormalities were uncovered, and she was discharged to go home.

What other data might be useful in following a patient in shock?

What other symptoms are common in a patient who is hypotensive?

How does anaphylaxis usually present in man?

Hypotension is a cardinal feature of a patient who is in shock, a state of circulatory insufficiency in which the vital organs are inadequately perfused. One usually monitors mentation as a measure of brain perfusion. A Foley catheter should have been inserted in this patient's bladder to aid in monitoring her course.

Conscious hypotensive patients frequently complain of thirst or shortness of breath or gastrointestinal symptoms such as a sense of an impending bowel movement. They are often confused or agitated and may be very difficult to deal with. The combative patient may be in shock and should not be written off as a behavior problem. It is essential to know hematocrit, BUN, electrolytes, urinary flow, and central venous pressure in dealing with such a patient.

Anaphylaxis in man is usually a respiratory syndrome with laryngeal edema or wheezing. A rash is common, and the syndrome almost always follows parenteral injection, commonly of penicillin. If indeed this patient had an anaphylactic reaction to ampicillin, it was unusual in two regards. It followed a single oral dose (she had taken the drug in the past with no ill effects), and it led to hypotension with no obvious respiratory involvement. The mechanism of anaphylaxis begins with an antigen-antibody reaction followed by release of intermediate mediators such as histamine, serotonin, slow-reacting substance, and bradykinin. Shock may be caused by a low cardiac output in the face of a high arteriolar resistance and a shifting of fluid from the intravascular compartment to the intracellular or extracellular-extravascular spaces. Presumably the selection of the blood vessels instead of the lungs as a "shock organ" is the result of the precise combination of intermediate agents in this specific patient.

The unusual response to epinephrine remains unexplained. Corticosteroids should probably have been given in the ER, but their action is not immediate, and deferring such therapy was probably not harmful. Epinephrine may be given in doses up to 1 mg intravenously and that repeatedly, generally with no ill effects. Subcutaneous or even intramuscular injections should be avoided in a hypotensive patient, since perfusion to skin and muscle may be inadequate. The drug would then not be picked up until much later.

This case was never well understood by the physicians involved, but fortunately the patient recovered.

61

A 2-YEAR-OLD BOY was brought to the ER by his concerned parents because he seemed unduly sleepy and had vomited several times. Three hours earlier he had fallen off the top bunk of a double bunk bed, landing on his right side and hitting the right side of his head.

On arrival in the ER, he seemed alert and would cry vigorously if stimulated. He could walk well and move all extremities well, had equal and reactive pupils, and had no facial or head abnormalities. He had no evidence of other injuries and had made no prior visits to the ER for injuries. A skull series of x-rays was done; they were unremarkable.

How unusual is it for children to vomit after head injuries?

Should arteriography be done?

Is this a case of a "battered child"?

What are the usual features of a case of child battering?

Although vomiting is a serious symptom in an adult with head injury, it is of less diagnostic significance in a child, since it is present in a high percentage of children with relatively trivial head injuries. This child, like all others with head injury, needs careful observation over the ensuing twenty-four hours. He should be watched for arousability and the development of gross focal neurologic defects. Since he has a responsible family, we will send him home with careful instructions. We tell the parents to wake him every two hours and walk him to the bathroom. If he can do this highly coordinated maneuver with ease, he has been adequately observed and can go back to bed for two more hours. An alarm clock must be set at two-hour intervals. This is far more valuable and less dangerous than an arteriogram. Of course, if he deteriorates, he must be returned to the ER and studied further.

This case is probably not one of parental abuse. Only one feature, the situation of a fall from the top bunk, suggests it. Child abuse or "child battering" may account for up to 30% of fractures, burns, and head injuries in young children. The physician's suspicions should be aroused by an injury that is inconsistent with the reported trauma; an inordinate delay in bringing the child to medical attention; prior injuries to the child or a sibling; the child's failure to thrive; and bizarre injuries (in this case for example, one must ask what a 2-year-old child was doing on a top bunk).

Parents of battered children usually have a history of beating for discipline, but they rarely use one medical facility regularly. There may be a family crisis, perhaps a very small one, and no source of help, and the parents take out their hostility on the child. The presence of retinal hemorrhages in a young child is almost diagnostic of severe head trauma. Long-bone x-rays and skull films often reveal many new and old fractures. It is usually not a good idea for the ER physician to accuse the family of child abuse. We urge early involvement of the pediatrics resident or senior staff physician. The child may need hospitalization for protection even if this is not warranted by the severity of his injuries.

The physician may either feel contempt for the injured child's family or despair of effecting any change in their treatment of the child, but neither attitude is warranted. Child-battering parents were usually battered or neglected children themselves, and only by supporting and encouraging them can agencies help them change their pattern of child-rearing. The physician's hostility may drive them "underground" and thus away from sources of help to which the pediatrics department might refer them.

A 20-YEAR-OLD WOMAN in an angry and disheveled state was
brought to the ER by the police. She had been in the ER several
times in the preceding two weeks and had been difficult to deal with.
On this occasion she appeared well except for her obvious belligerence,
ataxia, slurred speech, and tendency to go to sleep if undisturbed.
She smelled of alcohol and had been arrested by the police for
being drunk in a public place. She was on a "drunk hold" and thus
was handcuffed to her bed.

The physician who examined her believed that she was intoxicated.
When asked what should be done with her, he said in a loud voice
that "someone ought to take her out and shoot her." Overhearing
this, several other patients became very distressed. One nurse made
a deprecating comment about interns. The patient was sober enough
to walk in about four hours, and she was discharged to the city jail.

What is a "hold"?

Does good bedside manner preclude any specific sort of comments?

The term *hold* in our ER does not refer to wrestling. A police arrest is termed a *hold* and may be of several types. A *mental health hold* is placed on someone whose bizarre behavior and speech arouse in the arresting officer suspicion of mental illness. Such a hold can be dropped without the patient's being booked after any physician has seen the patient. We usually ask our psychiatry team to see such a patient with us.

A *drunk hold* is an arrest for a crime — usually being drunk in a public place. Such a patient usually gets a medical evaluation but is still under arrest for a crime. If the police diagnosis is erroneous (e.g., the patient turns out to be hypoglycemic), the hold may be dropped, but only if it is not yet entered in the police log book. Other hold patients who have been arrested and imprisoned in city or county jails will be seen in our ER. While with us, these patients are the responsibility of the county sheriffs' deputies stationed in the ER. The prisoners are housed in the ER jail cell or shackled to their beds. Infrequently, they try to escape, and the deputies appreciate our not aiding or abetting the prisoners, however unintentionally. The physician must fill out a special jail medical form before a jail patient returns to prison. He should be very complete and specific in his instructions on this form, because jail attendants are not permitted to do more or less than the physician's orders specify.

In this case, the physician's comment obviously was in poor taste and totally unlike his usual approach to patients. It should have served as a signal to him and others that it was time for a coffee break.

A physician's bedside manner is very much his own. Each physician develops his own approach. There is almost nothing that cannot be said to a patient if he is convinced of his physician's interest and good will. In a good relationship, a patient may be reassured by statements as bold as "you have a 50–50 chance of making it through to tomorrow." However, we often deal in inadequately developed doctor-patient relationships in which one must be more careful. In addition, the ER is not very private, and observers may react vigorously and negatively to what they believe is the staff's disrespectful behavior to patients.

A 17-YEAR-OLD WOMAN came to the ER complaining of vaginal spotting since four hours earlier that morning. She was four months pregnant and had already been seen twice in the obstetrics clinic. This was her first pregnancy, and she very much wanted the baby. Early in the pregnancy she had suffered with nausea and vomiting; otherwise, she was well. Her past history was uneventful except for an allergy to penicillin. This day she had lost about two teaspoonfuls of blood vaginally and was quite concerned.

The examining physician found the patient on a bed holding tightly to her young husband's hand. Her vital signs included blood pressure 120/72 supine and 110/50 seated, pulse 80 supine or seated, and temperature 36.2°C orally. Head, eyes, and throat were normal. Her chest was clear. Her abdomen showed slight tenderness throughout and a uterus halfway between pubis and umbilicus. A pelvic exam by speculum was done and disclosed a blue cervix with a closed os. There was no inordinate tenderness.

How often does bleeding occur in pregnancy?

Is it ever dangerous to do a pelvic exam in such a setting?

What is wrong with this young woman, and what should be done?

Bleeding is common in pregnancy, occurring in perhaps a third of pregnancies, even those that go on to a healthy, full-term delivery. The significance of the bleeding varies depending on the stage of pregnancy.

We see a fair number of women with incomplete abortions in the first trimester. Such patients will have significant bleeding, usually more than their usual quantity for a menstrual period, or will pass actual tissue other than blood. We examine such a patient and, if the os is open wide, usually explore the uterus. This is done by the on-call gynecologist on the following basis: If the uterus is less than twelve weeks' size and no evidence of sepsis is present, the uterus is explored immediately after the diagnosis of incomplete abortion is established. This exploration includes removal of placental fragments with a sponge forceps or large currette or suction uterine aspirator. No dilation is carried out, since the cervix already is open. However, occasionally some sedation, such as Demerol or Valium, may be necessary. If the patient is accompanied by a friend or relative, she may receive sedation and be sent home without admission. The usual routine is to send the patient home following uterine exploration, with careful instructions regarding followup.

This procedure should not be confused with a D. and C. It is simply an instrumental exploration of the uterus, without dilation of the cervix, and requires no anesthesia. It will cut down blood loss and morbidity if done immediately. Any evidence of infection or excessive blood loss detected by the resident requires admission.

Once into the second trimester, abortions are much less frequent. This patient probably has less than a 10% chance of completing an abortion. She is said to have a threatened abortion and will be reassured and sent home. She should be told to return if she begins to pass copious amounts (more than enough to use one sanitary pad per hour) of blood or tissue or to have severe pain. She should avoid intercourse and douching (no douching ever during pregnancy). She should be seen again in any case at the obstetrics clinic within one month.

If bleeding occurs in the last half of the pregnancy, we advise not doing a pelvic exam in the emergency department. A placenta praevia or abruptio may be present, and examination might increase the chance of losing the fetus. Of course, copious bleeding may require us to start several intravenous routes, give quantities of fluid, and type and crossmatch and perhaps transfuse many units of blood. If the patient is hemorrhaging vigorously, her life takes precedence and a pelvic exam should be done. Sometimes the products of conception are found in the cervical os, and simple removal quiets down the bleeding.

When the bleeding is so severe as to force a pelvic exam, it should, of course, begin with a careful speculum examination, which has less chance than a bimanual exam of disturbing a placenta praevia. Ultrasound too is available and useful in diagnosing such pathology as placenta praevia.

The thoroughness of the physician's examination, his explanation of the patient's symptoms, and his reassurance that her pregnancy is a normal one are most important here. It is not enough for the physician to assure *himself* that nothing is wrong; he must convey this feeling to the woman, also.

64

A 52-YEAR-OLD MAN came to the ER complaining of difficulty getting his breath. He had been troubled with shortness of breath fairly badly for the past two weeks, but it had become even worse today. He said that he had asthma.

The man had smoked two packs of cigarettes a day for many years and had a total smoking history of over sixty pack-years. He had quit smoking six months earlier when he was discharged from the state penitentiary where he had been a prisoner for nine years. He did not wish to discuss the cause of his incarceration. Shortness of breath had become noticeable about age 40 and was more and more frequently a problem during the past year. He had been told while in prison that he had asthma and had been treated with a combination drug containing ephedrine, theophylline, and barbiturate. At times he had been on corticosteroids and used an isoproterenol inhaler.

During the past two years the patient had been bothered by a cough usually productive of a few ounces of yellow sputum daily. In fact, when pressed, he admitted to a "cigarette cough" most mornings of the past ten years. The cough was worse in the past few days, and the sputum was becoming darker, a sort of grayish green in color. During the past six months he had never been free of cough and could never walk more than three blocks without having to stop to get his breath. The preceding night he was up most of the night with coughing and difficulty getting his breath.

On examination the patient was observed to be obviously having some difficulty breathing. He appeared fatigued and could say no more than a few words at a time between breaths. His chest was hyperexpanded, and he took a long time with each breath. Vital signs included blood pressure 160/90, pulse 90, respiration 24, jugular venous pressure elevated in expiration but normal in inspiration, and temperature 37.0°C orally. His breath sounds were altered: One could not hear any normal alveolar breath sounds, but he did have high-pitched wheezes bilaterally. His heart was best heard in the epigastrium, and the heart tones were normal. His liver was low, with an upper edge percussible at almost the costal margin but with a total height in the midclavicular line of only 11 centimeters. There was no edema, and the rest of the examination showed no abnormalities.

Does this man have asthma?

What sort of problems lead to the appearance of such a patient at the emergency room doors?

What can be done for him in the ER?

Most middle-aged or older patients who arrive at the ER with the comment that their asthma is getting worse do not have asthma. A few of them have severe congestive heart failure, even pulmonary edema. These can often be diagnosed by the presence of edema, hepatomegaly, and above all an elevated venous pressure. These patients with pulmonary edema may have no rales but rather a chest full of musical wheezes, hence the term "cardiac asthma." The history may include episodes of paroxysmal nocturnal dyspnea occurring two to four hours after going to bed, aiding diagnosis.

More often, as in this case, the older patient who labels himself as asthmatic has a chronic obstructive lung disease of the emphysema-bronchitis type. He may present with a history primarily of dyspnea for many years, may be oxygenated but wasted, and can be described as a "pink puffer." Such a patient usually can be kept out of the hospital until his ultimate decline and thus never accumulates a large inpatient chart. He has been said to have a "negative New York City telephone book sign" (his inpatient chart is less thick than the NYC telephone book). The patient suffering from relatively pure emphysema is less common than the bronchitic patient who describes years of cough before he developed significant dyspnea and appears more flushed but often cyanotic. This "blue bloater" arrives frequently at the ER with the complications of infection (worsening bronchitis, pneumonia, or bronchiolitis), heart failure, mechanical disasters (pneumothorax, enlarging bleb restricting the vital capacity), or pulmonary emboli. Such a patient thus has many hospital admissions, with a consequent "positive NYC telephone book sign."

The patient described has characteristics both of emphysema and of bronchitis. He may also have some airway narrowing that will respond to bronchodilators and is therefore termed reversible. We treat him in the ER with low-flow oxygen and intravenous infusion of 500 mg of aminophylline in 500 ml of 5% dextrose in water, and obtain lab data including CBC, chest x-ray, ECG, and arterial blood gases. We look at the sputum but seldom find it helpful to culture it unless the chest x-ray defines a pneumonia. Occasionally we can discharge such a patient on antibiotics (we prefer tetracycline or ampicillin), but usually we are obliged to admit him for further evaluation and therapy. It is difficult to get a patient to do the most important bronchial toilet activities at home until he has been taught and observed doing these in the hospital.

65

A 33-YEAR-OLD MAN was brought to the ER by ambulance. He had been despondent and had attempted suicide by shooting himself with a .38-caliber revolver. The bullet entered two intercostal spaces below the left nipple and exited at the left posterior axillary line in the tenth intercostal space.

On arrival at the ER the patient was conscious and breathing. He had a palpable systolic blood pressure of 60 mm Hg. His cardiac rate was 130 per minute. Three large intravenous infusions were begun with lactated Ringer's solution. A right internal jugular line and two antecubital fossa lines were placed with large-diameter short intracatheters. Within five minutes 500 ml of fluid had been given, and his blood pressure was palpable and audible at 100 mm Hg. A single chest tube was placed in the left midaxillary line in the fifth interspace. The pectoralis major muscle was grasped and the tube placed just posterior to it. The tube was connected to underwater drainage and then via a three-bottle system to continuous suction. Less than 100 ml of blood returned via the chest tube.

A Foley indwelling bladder catheter and a nasogastric tube were placed. A portable chest x-ray was taken. It showed a normal chest and a metal fragment probably below the diaphragm. The patient was told he needed an operation, and within thirty minutes of his arrival at the ER he was moved into the operating room. At that time the central venous pressure readings from his jugular vein catheter were about 14 centimeters. Eight units of blood were readied, he was intubated and anesthetized, and his abdomen was opened.

The laparotomy exposed about 1000 ml of free blood in the peritoneal cavity, a bisected spleen, and tears in the stomach and the jejunum. As the spleen was being removed, the patient's blood pressure became unobtainable despite a CVP of 18 centimeters.

The chest was then opened, and a bulging pericardium was incised. A large amount of clot was easily evacuated, and a tangential crease wound of the apex of the heart was reinforced with sutures. The blood pressure rose on opening the pericardium, and the rest of the operation proceeded uneventfully.

When and how should chest tubes be placed?

When should a traumatized patient have his chest opened in the ER?

Is there any value to needle pericardiocentesis in a traumatic hemopericardium?

We feel rather free to place chest tubes. Any traumatized patient who is dyspneic, tachypneic, or hypotensive or anyone in whom we clinically suspect a pneumothorax or hemothorax usually gets one or two chest tubes placed even before the five minutes it would take to obtain a portable x-ray of the chest. Physical findings of the chest may be nonrevealing and easily confused. A serious hemothorax may be missed by relying on auscultation. Chest tubes are fairly benign considering the tremendous potential danger of the patient's basic problems.

Usually we prefer two tubes, an anterior one in the second or third intercostal space at the midclavicular line and a posterior one at the midaxillary line and sixth or seventh intercostal space directed posteriorly. If the patient is awake, we try to anesthetize the skin and perichondrium with about 10 ml of 1% lidocaine, make a stab wound in the skin, separate deeper layers down to and including the parietal pleura with a large clamp or spreading movements of a pair of scissors, and then probe the wound with a gloved finger. If the finger tells you that you are in the chest, a large chest tube is placed by grasping its tip in a large curved surgical clamp and advancing it over your probing finger. Tubes have been mistakenly placed below the diaphragm. This does no good and may damage liver or spleen, so we try to avoid it. Occasionally we use a single tube placed as in this case. It is not uncommon for chest tubes to be placed on the wrong side (appearing correct until it is observed that the bullet's trajectory was bizarre and led to contralateral damage). If in doubt or if the patient is not improving, we do not hesitate to place two tubes on the other side.

Whenever a patient has sustained chest trauma and is being re-suscitated with closed chest massage that still fails to produce a palpable pulse, we urge opening the chest. Needle pericardiocentesis is of very little value. It usually returns nothing even when much blood has clotted in the pericardium and led to cardiac tamponade. Search for a paradoxical pulse is also useless. This sign, defined in a spontaneously breathing patient with resting respiration, is grossly distorted in a patient who is in respiratory distress and totally obviated in one who is receiving positive pressure ventilation. The only useful signs are hypotension and a high or rising central venous pressure. It is not impossible to plug a myocardial rent with a finger and place a few sutures in the ER as a holding maneuver until the operating room's greater resources can be reached. In this most dramatic situation, one who hesitates is lost. Hypotension following chest trauma may be due to cardiac tamponade and after a brief but vigorous search for other sources of blood loss, the heart should be attacked directly. Sometimes this must be done in the ER.

In this case the initial approach failed to turn up an intrathoracic cause for the patient's hypotension. The next obvious place to look was his abdomen, and it was quickly opened. However, the more serious disturbance was intrathoracic, and it was treated appropriately. If he had not responded promptly in the ER, a thoracotomy could have been done there. Nevertheless, the best place for these maneuvers is still a well-equipped and well-lighted operating room. Optimally, the patient should have been taken directly to the operating room for resuscitation.

66

A 65-YEAR-OLD MAN came to the ER complaining of chest pain. He said the pain in his right side had begun about twenty-four hours earlier and had been getting worse since then. It was constantly present but excruciating when he coughed or moved suddenly. He was most comfortable sitting quietly or lying on his right side. Although he denied smoking or drinking, he did admit to a cough the preceding few days that produced a small amount of yellow sputum. Prior to this illness he had been quite well and active and denied any chronic cough, prior chest pains, or shortness of breath.

On physical examination the patient appeared well. His vital signs included blood pressure 150/80, pulse 100, respiration 20, temperature 38.3°C orally, and a normal jugular venous pressure. His head, eyes, ears, nose, and throat were unremarkable. His neck was carefully palpated, revealing no adenopathy or other pathology. His chest was slightly tender laterally on the right side, and there were a few crackling rales audible there. His cardiovascular examination was normal; he had no edema; and the rest of the exam showed nothing remarkable. A chest x-ray showed a right lower lobe infiltrate involving almost the entire lobe.

What is the diagnosis in this case?

What further studies should be done?

What should be done for this man?

This man seems to have a pneumonia, and most pneumonias are pneumococcal. Indeed, this is the usual organism no matter what the host situation. Alcoholics, postinfluenza patients, diabetics, and the like, all usually have the pneumococcus as causative organism when they develop a bacterial pneumonia.

We recommend obtaining blood samples for arterial blood-gas analysis, also CBC, blood culture, and a sputum sample for culture and for gram stain. The sputum smear should be examined by the requesting physician and will probably show a preponderance of one organism. If this is indeed a gram-positive diplococcus, therapy should be begun with penicillin. Care must be taken in obtaining the sputum (not saliva). This patient (if not allergic to penicillin) could be given 2.4 million units of procaine penicillin G intramuscularly followed by 500 mg of penicillin V orally qid.

Because our bed capacity is limited, we often are not able to admit patients with pneumonia to the hospital. Many do well at home. A diffuse bronchopneumonia in a young patient may be treated with tetracycline or erythromycin, 500 mg qid. A patient with lobar pneumonia should get penicillin as described. These outpatient regimens need careful monitoring. The patient must return in two or three days, sooner if he is worse. The patients who have lowered host resistance or appear very ill should be admitted to the hospital. Any alcoholic with pneumonia needs hospitalization. Similarly, a seizure patient or a diabetic should be admitted. Most patients over age 50 should be admitted. The presence of a high fever, tachypnea, severe chest pain, or hypoxia argues for admission. In Denver a normal arterial pO_2 may be as low as 65 mm Hg, leaving little room for worsening.

This patient was treated at home, and he improved rapidly. When seen again in three days, he felt much better and was afebrile. In two weeks his chest x-ray was normal and he had returned to normal.

67

A 38-YEAR-OLD MAN was brought to the emergency room by city police. He had been arrested for being drunk in a public place and taken to the city jail. After seven hours in jail he had appeared "too drunk" to his jailers and was brought to the ER. Because no ER beds were available, the man was placed in the locked ER jail cell. A physician saw him within one hour of his arrival in the ER but quickly turned away. The patient was disheveled, malodorous, uncooperative, unshaven, ataxic, and appeared quite drunk. No careful neurologic or mental status exam was done, and he was left in the cell to sober up. When next seen three hours later, he was stuporous and had one large pupil. He was quickly taken from the cell, undressed, examined, and rushed to the operating room, where an epidural hematoma was evacuated. Despite these vigorous efforts the patient died on the operating table.

How can you tell that a patient is drunk?

How can you tell that he is *just* drunk?

Is it surprising that this man had no obvious signs of trauma and yet had an acute epidural hematoma?

Does an acute subdural hematoma also present this way?

Although alcohol intoxication is a common pathologic state in most ERs, it is frequently misdiagnosed. The features that should be looked for include slurred speech, a tendency to drift off to sleep, inappropriate behavior, and mild ataxia. A blood alcohol is helpful. A level of 100 mg per 100 ml is used in most states to define a patient as too drunk to drive; one is usually definitely ataxic at 200 mg per 100 ml, and stupor appears at about 300 mg per 100 ml in the occasional drinker. A chronic alcoholic (the "chronic" is redundant) may not become sleepy until a higher level — 400 or 500 mg per 100 ml — due to CNS tolerance to the alcohol. In this patient, who had been off alcohol for at least eight hours when first seen in the ER, a blood alcohol probably would have been under 100 mg per 100 milliliters. Such a low level would have alerted the physician to the presence of another problem.

The big problem is ruling out the existence of other pathology accompanying alcohol intoxication as cause of the ataxia or stupor. This patient was still "drunk" after seven hours of sobering up time, and the physician should have made a more careful search for other pathology. A patient with a blood alcohol of 400 mg per 100 ml may also have a subdural hematoma, an epidural hematoma, cerebellar degeneration, or any other pathology. The examination should include vital signs (a wide pulse pressure or bradycardia may be the tip-off to rising CSF pressure), gait, mentation, and a careful search for head trauma. It is very difficult to evaluate CNS disorders in a drunk patient.

It is not surprising that there was no gross evidence of head trauma. Epidural hematomas often result from a relatively small trauma that hits at precisely the right spot to tear the middle meningeal artery. A baseball or hockey puck can do this. The patient with an acute subdural hematoma is more often the victim of more massive trauma: He was hit by a car or a truck rather than a baseball. As a result, he has multiple injuries, and since focal neurologic signs may be scant, we sometimes spend valuable time elsewhere before evaluating the cause of his confusion or unconsciousness. A chronic subdural hematoma often presents weeks after the trauma, and the patient may no longer give a history of any trauma. This disorder is replacing syphilis as "the great imitator" and should be thought of in any confused or sleepy patient. This is especially true if he is aged or an alcoholic, frequent settings for a chronic subdural hematoma.

68

A 30-YEAR-OLD MAN was brought to the emergency room by ambulance. He had reportedly held up three small stores that evening and had been caught by the police as he was making his escape from the third robbery. The police ordered him to stop, fired a warning shot, and finally fired a shot that entered his thorax just to the left of the fourth thoracic vertebra and exited anteriorly next to the sternum. No resuscitative measures were carried out for the fifteen minutes between the shooting and the man's arrival in the ER. On arrival he was pulseless and had no respiration. His pupils were fixed and dilated. The patient was declared dead after a brief attempt at resuscitation. He was said to be a known narcotics addict with many arrests for theft and other offenses. His body was covered and placed in a room in the back of the emergency department.

Thirty minutes later the parents of this patient had been found by the police and were brought to the ER. They were told of their son's death by a physician. They responded with no show of grief and said they knew it would end like this some day. The parents were asked to stay to speak with a coroner, but he was delayed and they went home an hour later. At no time were the parents asked to identify the body, nor did they ask to see it, despite the fact that it was only 20 feet from the room they were in.

Two hours later a pair of detectives came to speak to the ER physician. They said they had viewed the body and that it was not that of the man previously named. The physician immediately realized that he did not know whether the correct family had been notified of the death of their son. Attempts to find either family were unsuccessful until the next day.

What is the responsibility of the ER physician to the next of kin?

Would the ER physician be liable for results of this misinformation?

Fortunately — although the body and also the family that was notified were both misidentified in this case — by chance they paired correctly and the dead man did belong to the family that came to the ER. A mistaken middle initial had led to the confusion. The ER or the coroner's staff should insist on the family identifying the body. This could have been a grievous error, for which the ER physician would have been entirely responsible. The emergency-room physician should be aware of the need for identification. The physician should also assume the role of physician to the next of kin, allowing them to express their sadness and providing whatever comforts and privacy are available.

69[*]

69 [*]

A 45-YEAR-OLD MAN arrived at the emergency room complaining of dyspnea. His temperature was 38.8°C and he had diffuse bilateral wheezes. His chest x-ray was clear with no infiltrate. There was no evidence of congestive heart failure, nor did any show up on physical examination. The man had a left ventricular heave and apical systolic murmur. He stated that he was a patient at the cardiac clinic and was on propranolol (Inderal) for repeated episodes of rapid heartbeat but was not on any digitalis preparation. He was thought to have an acute bronchitis, and therapy was begun with isoproterenol (Isuprel).

A second physician arrived and curtailed the isoproterenol therapy. He suspected that a patient being treated for tachyarrhythmia with propranolol but no digitalis might have subaortic stenosis. The patient's hospital chart was obtained; it carried the diagnosis of idiopathic hypertrophic subaortic stenosis and noted that the patient had a strong adverse reaction to beta adrenergic agents. Therapy for his bronchitis was continued with very low dosage aminophylline plus corticosteroids and antibiotics.

Why is it important to avoid beta adrenergic agents in this case?

How can the diagnosis be made more available in emergencies such as this?

*Adapted from Platt, F. W., Look out for a rare bird. *Emergency Medicine* 4:73, April 1972. Used by permission of the publisher.

Idiopathic hypertrophic subaortic stenosis is a rare disorder. However, it is one physicians should be familiar with because of the seemingly paradoxical responses to beta adrenergic agents and those drugs that increase cardiac muscle contraction. The effect of aminophylline on the heart is variable, but it can be considered a weak beta adrenergic agent in contrast to isoproterenol and epinephrine. These much stronger beta adrenergic agents are contraindicated in this condition because they increase the muscular obstruction to the left ventricle outflow tract.

The diagnosis is difficult to make but once made should be explained to the patient, noted for an examining physician on an identifying bracelet or necklace, and noted in any hospital records on the patient. One should suspect such a diagnosis when a patient is on an unusually discrepant program of drug therapy. For example, it should be suspected if he has obvious angina pectoris but is not being treated with nitroglycerin, or if he has runs of tachyarrhythmia or congestive heart failure but is not being treated with digitalis. Patients with diabetes, patients on anticoagulant therapy or corticosteroids, and patients with strong allergic reactions to any drugs should wear such identifying bracelets.

70 *

A 34-YEAR-OLD MAN collapsed just outside the emergency department. His friend told of a three-day course of progressive cough and fatigue. The patient had been well previously and was not on special drugs. He was hypotensive, grossly cyanotic, and had a sinus tachycardia of 140 beats per minute. His breathing was shallow at about 30 respirations per minute, and he had bilateral rales and rhonchi. His venous pressure was not elevated, and he had no edema. Oxygen therapy was begun but held to 4 liters per minute because the attending physician was concerned about the possible danger of high-flow oxygen. An arterial blood sample showed a pO_2 of 40 mm Hg that produced a saturation of less than 70%. A chest film showed multiple large infiltrates thought to be pneumonia. Increasing the nasal oxygen flow to 12 liters per minute raised the oxygen saturation to 80%.

How much oxygen does one give a patient?

*Adapted from Platt, F. W., Enough is not too much. *Emergency Medicine* 4:46, February 1972. Used by permission of the publisher.

The critical factor in oxygen therapy is to give enough oxygen. Even though there are those patients with chronic obstructive lung disease who cannot tolerate uncontrolled high-flow oxygen, they need high-flow oxygen, perhaps with the use of a ventilator. Oxygen therapy should never be withheld or kept to a low flow when the patient is still hypoxic simply because the physician is afraid of giving too much oxygen.

We see similar reluctance to give enough of an appropriate therapy in many situations. Patients in shock are given inadequate volumes of intravenous fluids, agitated withdrawing alcoholics are given too little sedation, and patients in pain are given too little analgesia. Too much of a good thing may be bad, but too little is terrible.

71*

A 20-YEAR-OLD WOMAN came to the emergency room after she had taken 20 to 30 Anacin tablets and an unknown quantity of iron capsules. She had already vomited spontaneously and appeared somewhat anxious. Since her physical exam revealed nothing unusual, she was observed for two hours and sent home. She returned the next day confused and complaining of persistent vomiting and hematemesis. Her stomach was distended and contained over 1500 ml of bloody material. In addition, she was hypotensive — her reclining blood pressure was 90/60 and dropped 20 mm when she sat up. Her BUN was 48 mg per 100 milliliters. The patient was admitted to the hospital, and she improved with subsequent care.

What was the problem here?

What other drugs are more dangerous than would be initially apparent when taken in overdoses?

*Adapted from Platt, F. W., Ironclad problem. *Emergency Medicine* 4:165, January 1972. Used by permission of the publisher.

The severity of aspirin and iron intoxication in adults is often underestimated. The danger cannot be measured in terms of coma, as it can after the ingestion of many other, more common substances. Iron can produce a severe hemorrhagic gastritis that can lead to death. Aspirin produces a series of severe metabolic disturbances that may culminate in a metabolic acidosis or a respiratory alkalosis. Both of these ingestions require thorough initial evaluation and vigorous therapy. This should include arterial blood-gas studies and other evaluations of the patient's metabolic status before discharge.

The other drug overdoses we most often see underappreciated in our ER are the antidepressants, which may well present with a conscious patient and yet lead to fatal arrhythmias.

72

A 55-YEAR-OLD MAN was brought to the emergency room by ambulance. He was complaining of abdominal pain. As he was wheeled into the ER, the ambulance attendant mentioned that he had been unable to feel a pulse. The patient was immediately surrounded by a group of physicians and nurses, who noted that he was apparently conscious and communicating but indeed had no obtainable blood pressure and no obtainable peripheral pulses. His carotid pulse was palpable and his heart rate 110. There were several long scars on his chest, abdomen, and legs. An electrocardiogram showed a broad QRS with a duration of 0.16 second and a regular rate of 110. No P waves were evident. A central venous pressure line was placed, and it read 28 centimeters. The physician's initial impression was probably tempered by his just having been involved in a case of dissecting aortic aneurysm in which the diagnosis had initially been missed. It was difficult to avoid the same diagnosis in this case.

A call to the patient's regular physician revealed that this man had undergone extensive vascular surgery including myocardial revascularization in the past two years. He had shown no palpable pulses for many months. The ECG was then reviewed, and the diagnosis of hyperkalemia was made. Therapy was begun with glucose, insulin, and sodium bicarbonate. Serum potassium level was 6.8 mEq per liter.

What is the usual first therapy given to a pulseless patient?

What are the ECG findings of hyperkalemia?

What are the usual causes of hyperkalemia?

A pulseless patient usually is assumed to be in ventricular fibrillation and greeted immediately with a direct current shock of 400 watt seconds even before a diagnostic ECG. Occasionally such a patient will be in severe shock, and there is indeed a possibility that the defibrillation will result in fibrillation rather than cure it. Even more rarely, as in this case, the pulseless patient will show evidence of adequate cardiac output (such as retaining consciousness), leading us to defer electroshock.

Hyperkalemia usually first leads to peaked T waves and lengthening of the PR interval. More severe hyperkalemia may cause loss of P wave (the atria develop an "atrial squirm"), widening of the QRS, and eventually a sine wave pattern easily mistaken for ventricular flutter or tachycardia. Hyperkalemia has two main causes: acidosis or uremia. This patient did indeed have renal failure, which led to both acidosis and uremia. Potassium therapy can of course worsen either of these.

73

A 19-YEAR-OLD WOMAN came to the emergency room requesting to be told whether she was pregnant. She said that her last menstrual period had been six weeks earlier and that she had not missed a period since she was 14 years old. She said periods began at age 13 and had occurred irregularly since then. However, she then admitted that the menses occurred about every twenty-six days but that by "irregular" she meant they started on a different date each month. She felt well but on questioning admitted that her breasts felt a bit full and that she was getting up at night to urinate, an unusual practice for her. She had not been on any form of birth control in the past but was unmarried and claimed not to want a child.

What is the usual cause of amenorrhea in a young woman?

What should be done for this patient in the ER?

Is there any need for urgency?

Amenorrhea in a young woman is almost always due to pregnancy and requires no emergency care unless other significant symptoms are associated. Severe vomiting in pregnancy may need therapy. The amenorrhea may really be due to a disease process if she has other symptoms.

We usually do not examine such a patient in the ER, although at this date some early signs of pregnancy might be found, such as a bluish cervix and an enlarged uterus. At six weeks after the last menses, a test for chorionic gonadotropin (Gravindex) will probably be positive if done on a urine specimen with a specific gravity over 1.010. The agglutination test for human chorionic gonadotropin (HCG) is not always accurate and is only presumptive evidence of pregnancy, with several causes of false positives. Careful, gentle questioning regarding sexual intercourse is often helpful.

The cause for urgency here is the patient's wish not to have a child. She needs counseling regarding available alternatives, including abortion. Although we urge no single route, we do want her to have a clear understanding of the alternatives before time forces her to an unsatisfactory decision. For this reason we make rapid referrals to the obstetrics clinic.

74

A 40-YEAR-OLD MAN was brought to the ER because he had been found lying on the street unconscious. Shortly after his arrival, he had a five-minute major motor seizure. He was lying on a cart in the hall while a room was being readied for him when he had the fit. He was observed by several patients as well as their relatives and friends, two persons from housekeeping, two clerks, a policeman, and a nurse. The consternation was considerable among this group. The nurse found a physician and urged him to give the patient an injection of 10 mg of diazepam (Valium), which she handed him. The injection went in as the seizure was ending, to the great relief of the many observers. The patient was then given a brief physical examination which disclosed only stupor with no focal neurologic findings. He then was given 120 mg of phenobarbital intramuscularly. One hour later he was arousable enough to tell his story. He told of a seizure disorder of many years' standing but said he had recently stopped taking his usual diphenylhydantoin to see what would happen.

When a patient has a seizure in the ER, how many has he probably had that day?

How do seizure patients present in the ER, and how should they be treated?

Usually a seizure patient who has a fit in the ER is having the second one for that day — the first one brought him to the ER. Thus therapy is usually but not always appropriate. Seizure patients arriving at the ER can be classified in four groups: (1) known seizure disorder, (2) alcoholic — withdrawal or rum fits, (3) status, by definition: repeated seizures without awakening in the interim, and (4) first seizure in an adult. In general, a blood sugar sample should always be obtained, as close to ictus as possible. In a person on medication, it is helpful to know his Dilantin and phenobarbital levels for drug control.

1. *Known seizure disorder.* Paradoxically a person with a known seizure disorder may have a breakthrough in his control; this may be spontaneous, associated with drug juggling, or associated with alcohol intake, phenothiazines, sleep deprivation, etc. Therapeutic Dilantin level, by gas chromatography, is 1 to 2 mg per 100 ml or 10 to 20 μg per ml (20 μg to 30 μg is associated with nystagmus; 30 μg to 40 μg with dysarthria and ataxia, i.e., "drunk-like state"; above 40 μg with drowsiness). A patient who ran out of medications a few days ago should be given a loading dose of his proper medications, e.g., 500 mg of Dilantin orally bid the first day, 500 mg the second day, then 100 mg tid.

2. *Alcoholic.* Withdrawal seizure may be associated with early alcohol withdrawal signs and symptoms such as tremulousness, anxiety, fever, sweating, tachycardia, focal hallucinations, etc. This may occur while the patient is still drinking but tapering off. Alcoholics commonly have as causes for their seizures cerebral scars following head trauma. We often treat seizures in alcoholics prophylactically by giving phenobarbital intramuscularly (usually 120 mg for a 70-kg adult) and placing on maintenance phenobarbital (i.e., 30 mg tid) until a clinic visit. There is little evidence that diphenylhydantoin helps a withdrawing alcoholic, and we usually do not use it. The term *rum fit* actually refers to withdrawal seizures and so is a misnomer.

3. *Status.* This is a life-threatening disorder. (a) Treat with intravenous Valium in repeated 10-mg boluses up to 60 mg (remember,

there is no such thing as a "Valium drip" — it is immiscible). (b) Alternatively, give amobarbital, 500 mg intravenously; repeat if seizure has not stopped in five minutes. (Note: Be prepared to intubate to support respirations; i.e., endotracheal tube, laryngoscope, anesthesiologist, and Ambu bag.) (c) One can always stop status with general anesthesia, usually barbiturate. (d) Valium and amytal stop the present seizure but do not prevent future seizures. We don't give Valium to someone who is not at that moment having a seizure. The patient not in seizure must be placed on prophylactic anticonvulsants (i.e., phenobarbital, 90 to 240 mg per day, and Dilantin, 300 to 500 mg per day). (e) Use of intravenous Dilantin, 1000 mg given over more than twenty minutes, is useful in some cases but is dangerous due to cardiac arrhythmias. This is best given while the patient is on a cardiac monitor. Beware the acidosis after a seizure as a bad setting in which to give intravenous Dilantin.

4. *First seizure in an adult.* (a) This is usually a good reason for admission and a full neurologic workup to determine cause (toximetabolic, tumor, cardiovascular, subarachnoid hemorrhage, infection, etc.). (b) A history is needed from observer and patient regarding: first, warnings (aura) — visual hallucinations, olfactory hallucinations (funny or unpleasant smells), feeling of familiarity or strangeness, sensations or jerking in limbs; and second, the seizure itself — lip-smacking, verbalization, head and eyes turning, focal limb-jerking, tongue-biting, incontinence, generalized seizure. (c) A postictal exam should be done: The sooner it is done the more likely it will be to disclose a deficit. Look for focal limb weakness, reflex preponderance, unilateral Babinski sign, dysphasic speech, in other words, any focal signs. (d) The ER workup while waiting should include analysis of blood sugar, electrolytes, and BUN; ECG; chest and skull x-rays; and toxicologic studies for agents such as scopolamine, propoxyphene, tricyclic antidepressants, etc.

A 3-YEAR-OLD BOY was brought to the ER by his parents. He had fallen off a slide about an hour earlier and hit his head. He initially cried vigorously and then calmed down. The parents were very worried. They mentioned that he was their first and only child.

On examination, the child moved all extremities well, cried lustily when stimulated, and had no focal neurologic abnormalities. His fundi were hard to examine, since he kept moving his eyes, but they seemed normal. There was a small tender swelling high on his forehead, but no blood was seen behind the ears or tympanic membranes.

Skull films were taken and read as normal. The physician seemed saddened by these findings and told the parents they were normal with a very negative affect. The parents became more worried but agreed to observe the child closely that night.

How should "negative findings" such as a normal skull x-ray be presented to patients and families?

In general, when do you take skull x-rays?

75 DISCUSSION

Normal findings are good news and should be announced as such. A patient should feel that his doctor is working for his health, not for his diseases. This physician could better have approached the parents with a statement such as: "I have good news for you. The x-rays are normal. Your boy does not have a skull fracture. I'm sure you are as happy as I am to know that."

Skull x-rays should be done following loss of consciousness due to trauma or if a skull fracture is otherwise suspected. We do not advise x-rays for obscure medical-legal reasons. In fact, cervical spine films may be more important in cases of head injury. Skull films are also helpful in all situations in which the mental status cannot be evaluated, the history suggests severe head trauma, or the physical findings are equivocal.

A 27-YEAR-OLD MAN was brought to the emergency room by a good friend of his who was a third-year medical student. The patient had been well until two hours earlier, when he was suddenly seized by severe pain in his left flank. He said that the pain was the worst he had ever experienced, that it came and went, and that he felt weak and nauseated when the pain was present. On his arrival at the ER, the pain had been absent for over half an hour, and he felt a bit embarrassed at being there. His friend had already done a urinalysis and reported seeing many white blood cells and bacteria in the urine. The patient was afebrile, and his physical examination revealed nothing noteworthy. His friend felt that the diagnosis was pyelonephritis and that antibiotics were indicated. However, review of the urinalysis by a staff physician showed red blood cells instead of white blood cells.

What is the diagnosis in this case?

Why the confusion in doing the urinalysis?

What should be done for this patient?

This patient probably had ureteral colic. The story of sudden, varying, severe flank pain associated with hematuria suggests the presence of a stone in the ureter. Otherwise well people may have episodes of ureteral colic, which is usually severe pain. The pain may be flank, groin, scrotal, or a combination of these. A woman may complain of vulva or vaginal pain. There is usually vesicle irritability with dysuria and frequency of urination when the stone is entering the bladder. This patient probably has passed the stone into his bladder at this time.

Mistaking red blood cells for white is not a difficult error for a neophyte examining an unstained urine sediment. The identification of bacteria is almost impossible in an unstained sediment. Dust, debris, and amorphous crystals commonly oscillate in brownian movement and simulate bacteria. Only a gram stain, or better still a urine culture, will identify bacteruria. Of course, obstructive urinary disease and infective urinary disease are closely associated. Significant bacteruria may be present, and a urine culture would be appropriate.

We do an intravenous pyelogram (IVP), give the patient fluids and analgesics, and send him home. Before sending him home we obtain a serum calcium, phosphorus, alkaline phosphatase, uric acid, BUN, and creatinine. If he is sent home, we tell him to strain his urine and return for urinalyses daily. If he has fever or chills, extravasation of dye, a stone over 6 mm in diameter in the renal pelvis, or a nonfunctioning (totally obstructed) kidney, we usually admit him to the hospital.

This patient had an IVP which was normal except for slight dilation of the collecting system on the left. His friend became very upset when he heard that no antibiotics were to be given. When they left, the patient was reassured and his friend very anxious.

A 55-YEAR-OLD MAN was brought to the emergency room one morning by ambulance. He had wakened at 5:30, his usual time, with severe low back and hip pain, which he mentioned to his wife before driving to work at 7:00. Shortly thereafter he collapsed at his desk, and an ambulance was called.

On arrival at the ER the patient was cold and drenched in sweat. He denied being a diabetic or taking any medications and kept complaining of his low back and now low abdominal pain. He had a faint pulse with a palpable systolic blood pressure at 50 mm Hg and a rate of 100. His respiratory rate was 24. Venous pressure was difficult to estimate, but a central venous catheter placed in the internal jugular vein shortly gave a reading of 20 centimeters. The man said that he had suffered two myocardial infarctions three years and two years earlier but denied chest pain, high abdominal pain, or high back pain. Nonetheless, an ECG was taken, and it showed very elevated ST segments and QS waves across the precordium as well as small Q waves in the inferior leads.

The patient's chest sounded clear, and a portable chest x-ray was normal. His abdomen was soft and nontender, and a portable cross-table abdominal x-ray was normal. Three large intravenous routes were placed, a catheter was placed in his bladder, a nasogastric tube was placed, and he was given nasal oxygen.

He was admitted to the coronary care unit, and the cardiac surgery team was alerted.

The admitting diagnoses were acute anterior myocardial infarction, cardiogenic shock, and abdominal pain and back pain of uncertain etiology.

In the coronary care unit another ECG was taken, which showed much less ST elevation. The patient's private physician had been contacted and asked to describe the most recent ECG, which was apparently the same as the one done in the coronary care unit. The patient's back pain became worse, and his abdomen suddenly became distended. One hour after arrival at the ER, he was taken to the operating room.

What is the diagnosis in this case?

Why was his central venous pressure so high?

What led to the initial diagnostic error?

This patient gives a convincing story and appearance for the diagnosis of a bleeding or dissecting abdominal aneurysm. Although other diagnoses are tenable, this was indeed the correct one (bleeding aneurysm) and was first made by the physician who met the patient on the ambulance dock.

The ECG abnormality was apparently partly artifactually induced and confused the diagnosis. Over and over, we find the ECG is more confusing than helpful, especially when it conflicts with the history or physical findings. Some have even suggested that the ECG has no place in an emergency room.

Once a patient is in shock, for whatever reason, coronary artery perfusion suffers, and evidence of cardiac ischemia may be present. This may include ECG evidence and signs of heart failure. The high central venous pressure (CVP) here probably represented secondary cardiac failure. However, CVP readings may be erroneous. We have had catheters wander up into the neck or out into the pleural space. A second chest x-ray should have been taken to check on CVP tube placement.

78

A 19-YEAR-OLD WOMAN was brought to the emergency room by ambulance. She had claimed to have ingested several drugs, and her family called the city police, who in turn requested the ambulance and insisted that she be taken to the hospital. The ambulance attendant added the fact that he had just come back from a trip to pick her up, a trip requested directly by the family and refused by the patient. On arrival at the emergency room she identified herself as a hospital employee and refused any therapy. She claimed to have taken several dozen 5-mg diazepam (Valium) tablets and several 65-mg propoxyphene (Darvon) capsules. She insisted that she would not consent to any therapy and was going home. When asked about depression, she said she wanted to die.

A brief physical examination showed normal vital signs. When the patient refused to cooperate, she was tied hand and foot to the bed, a rubber nasogastric tube was passed despite her uncooperativeness, and 30 ml of syrup of ipecac plus 500 ml of warm water were instilled in the stomach. The tube was removed and her arm restraints removed. Fifteen minutes later she vomited copious material which included pill and capsule fragments. After two hours of observation during which she remained alert, she was transferred to the care of the ER psychiatry unit.

Should a patient be tied down and treated despite her refusal to give consent for such therapy?

If she signed a form signifying that she was leaving against medical advice, would the ER staff be absolved of blame if she came to harm?

Is punitive nasogastric intubation a good idea in ingestion cases?

What alternatives are there to emesis in the initial therapy of ingestions?

The cardinal rule of consent in emergency care is never to defer emergency care for lack of patient or parental consent. This patient was depressed, suicidal, and possibly already somewhat drugged, and she was in no condition to make a sound decision for her future. Withholding or delaying therapy would have had potentially lethal results and would have been erroneous. Reasonable therapeutic restraint is always proper in the ER.

An "AMA" (against medical advice) form has little place in an emergency room. It confuses the staff and allows poor therapy to be excused. A patient who refuses care for minor problems should have his refusal noted on his chart with a clear statement of the explanation that was given to him. If it is an emergency, however, he should be restrained and treated. Most patients will become cooperative when they realize we will not take *no* for an answer. This patient's refusal to cooperate despite her struggles with nasogastric tube suggests considerable masochistic need on her part. There is no place in medicine for a punitive physician or punitive therapy. In this case a firm but concerned approach is essential. The patient is distressed, and the therapy is distressing to staff and patient alike.

Emesis is usually the best way to empty a stomach. It may be produced by use of syrup of ipecac, as in this case, or apomorphine. The latter drug is given intravenously or subcutaneously. It works very rapidly but has the disadvantage of being itself a depressant. We usually give 0.1 mg per kg of body weight subcutaneously and follow it, after emesis has taken place, with naloxone, 0.8 mg total subcutaneously.

A large-bore Ewald-type stomach tube can be used for lavage, and this is probably second best. At least 2000 ml of water should be used in the lavage attempt. We fill and empty the stomach repeatedly with 400-ml amounts of saline or tap water. A small-bore Levine nasogastric tube is of very little value in lavage as it will not return pill fragments.

Possibly even more valuable would be the administration of a slurry of charcoal. If both ipecac and charcoal are to be used, the charcoal must be held until vomiting has occurred, otherwise the charcoal will absorb the ipecac.

A cathartic should usually be administered after emesis or lavage to further decrease absorption of the ingested drug.

79

A 36-YEAR-OLD MAN fainted at his office and was brought to the ER by ambulance. When he arrived, he claimed to feel well and to be ready to return to work. He said that a bout of nervousness at work had apparently led him to pass out and that he had no other symptoms. However, a friend who had accompanied him to the hospital pointed out that at lunch one hour earlier the patient had complained of a severe pain in his upper midabdomen. The patient did then admit to a little stomach upset but no pain. He had never before suffered from pains of any sort, including heartburn, gas pains, or indigestion. He had never before had a similar spell of nervousness or faintness. He was on no drugs and was otherwise well. He drank only occasionally and did not smoke.

On physical examination, the patient was observed to be perspiring heavily. Blood pressure was 100/80 supine and 90/70 seated. The patient pointed out that his blood pressure was always low, although he didn't know the usual numbers. His pulse was 110 supine and unchanged when he sat up. There were no other remarkable findings. An intravenous infusion was started, and nasal oxygen was administered. An ECG was taken and read as normal. The physician caring for this patient felt that he probably had had a myocardial infarction and admitted him to the coronary care unit. No rectal exam had been done because of the admitting diagnosis in the ER.

What are the usual reasons for profuse diaphoresis?

What danger is there in doing a rectal exam when the patient has had a myocardial infarction?

What is the diagnosis in this case?

Diaphoresis usually means hypoglycemia, shock, extreme expenditure of energy such as in a laboring asthmatic, or a very hot environment. This patient was in a cool room and was neither dyspneic nor laboring to breath. A blood sugar was drawn, and 50 ml of 50% glucose solution was given intravenously in the emergency room. There was no change in his condition, and the blood sugar was later reported to be normal.

It has been shown that a gentle rectal exam imposes very little stress in the presence of a fresh myocardial infarction, and such an exam should be done. In this case the cause of the fainting, sweating, and borderline hypotension was not clear, and occult bleeding must be considered. Indeed, the patient passed a large black diarrheal stool two hours later, and the problem was clarified. His bleeding duodenal ulcer was easily managed, and he did well subsequently. No further evidence of a myocardial infarction ever appeared.

Patients frequently deny serious significance to their symptoms. Denial is understandable but should not mislead the physician. Indeed, the admitting physician in this case was sure that he was dealing with serious cardiovascular illness even though the exact diagnosis was uncertain.

80

A 34-YEAR-OLD PHYSICIAN came to the ER by private car. He arrived walking bent over with his left arm held before him flexed at the elbow. He said that he was having terrible pain in his left shoulder and that it had begun fifteen minutes earlier, just after he had thrown a 50-pound bag of wood chips in his backyard. This was the sixth time he had suffered such an episode.

On examination, once the patient's shirt was removed, he seemed in much distress and was somewhat pale and sweaty. His right shoulder curvature was more rounded than the left, and there was a bulge anteriorly on the left side. He could not move his upper arm and complained much of pain.

What is the diagnosis in this case?

Should x-rays be taken?

What can you do to relieve this patient?

This patient has a recurring anterior shoulder dislocation. He probably should have a shoulder capsule reconstruction to avoid further recurrences. At the present time the object is to reduce his dislocation. Although fractures are seldom emergencies, dislocations almost always are, since nerve and vascular supplies may be damaged. Pain is also often more severe in dislocations than in most fractures. We commonly see dislocated fingers, shoulders, and hips in the emergency room.

Although we always x-ray a dislocation when it is a first-time event, we usually do not wait to obtain x-rays on repeat cases. The likelihood of a fracture-dislocation being present is very little in this case.

We usually lay the patient supine on a cart with his injured shoulder and arm hanging down off the edge. This may give some relief, and steady downward traction on the arm will relocate the shoulder in some cases. We generally use intravenous diazepam (Valium) analgesia and then attempt to reduce the shoulder dislocation. This patient was given 10 mg of Valium intravenously. Then, a sheet about his torso was pulled to the right, a large towel about his upper arm pulled to the left, and gentle manipulation of the arm flexed at the elbow led to relocation of the shoulder.

Once a dislocation is reduced, the pain diminishes radically, and any analgesia present will have much more effect. The patient often goes to sleep, and we have to beware a respiratory arrest if a large dose of analgesic was given.

Index

The numbers in this index refer to case numbers rather than page numbers.

The numbers in this index refer to case numbers rather than page numbers.

The numbers in this index refer to case numbers rather than page numbers.